BXAC

What's in Your Blood & Why You Should Care

HOW TO CLEANSE AND DETOXIFY YOUR BLOOD FOR OPTIMUM HEALTH

Earl Mindell, RPh, MH, PhD
Gene Bruno, MS, MHS

APR - - 2019

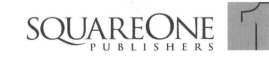

The information and advice contained in this book are based upon the research and the personal and professional experiences of the authors. They are not intended as a substitute for consulting with a healthcare professional. The publisher and authors are not responsible for any adverse effects or consequences resulting from the use of any of the suggestions, preparations, or procedures discussed in this book. All matters pertaining to your physical health should be supervised by a healthcare professional. It is a sign of wisdom, not cowardice, to seek a second or third opinion.

Cover Designer: Jeannie Rosado
In-House Editor: Michael Weatherhead
Typesetter: Gary A. Rosenberg

Square One Publishers
115 Herricks Road
Garden City Park, NY 11040
(516) 535-2010 • (877) 900-BOOK
www.squareonepublishers.com

Library of Congress Cataloging-in-Publication Data

Names: Mindell, Earl, author. | Bruno, Gene, author.
Title: What's in your blood & why you should care : how to cleanse & detoxify your blood for optimum health / Dr. Earl Mindell and Gene Bruno.
Other titles: What is in your blood and why you should care
Description: Garden City Park, NY : Square One Publishers, [2019] | Includes bibliographical references and index.
Identifiers: LCCN 2018049729 (print) | LCCN 2018051753 (ebook) | ISBN 9780757054433 (e-book) | ISBN 9780757004438 (pbk. : alk. paper)
Subjects: LCSH: Blood—Health aspects. | Diet therapy. | Detoxification (Health)
Classification: LCC QP91 (ebook) | LCC QP91 .M63 2019 (print) | DDC 612.1/1—dc23
LC record available at https://lccn.loc.gov/2018049729

Printed in the United States of America

10   9   8   7   6   5

Contents

Acknowledgments, iv

Introduction, 1

PART ONE

What You Need to Know About Your Blood

1. All About Your Blood, 5

2. What Your Blood Test Reveals, 25

3. How Your Body Cleanses Your Blood, 47

PART TWO

What Your Blood Needs

4. Understanding Nutrients, 63

5. Choosing Your Food, 87

6. Oxygen and Your Blood, 109

PART THREE

Detoxifying Your Blood

7. Foods and Fasts for Blood Cleansing, 127

8. Dietary Supplements That Support Detoxification, 143

9. Complementary Therapies, 165

Conclusion, 173

References, 175

About the Authors, 197

Index, 198

Acknowledgments

I would like to thank Rudy Shur, who always believes in important projects such as this one. I would also like to thank our editor, Michael Weatherhead, who was indispensable in completing this book. Finally, I would like to thank my wife, Gail; our children, Alanna and Evan; and our grandchildren, Lily and Ryan; for supporting my efforts on this book over the past year.

EM

The authorship of this book has been a journey—one that that was made possible with the help of a few key people, each of whom I would like to acknowledge. First, I would like to thank my publisher, Rudy Shur, who stood by me when my manuscript was more than just a little bit late. Second, I would like to thank my editor, Michael Weatherhead, who helped guide my words down better paths than would have been the case without his expert help. Finally, I would like to thank my wife, Kathy, and my son, Jameson, who supported my efforts even when it meant my taking time away from family life.

GB

Introduction

It is hard to deny that our modern environment is full of potentially harmful substances. At the same time, unless these toxins impact our lives in a very obvious and profound way—such as the toxic levels of lead found in the drinking water of Flint, Michigan—we tend not to give the matter too much thought. The unfortunate reality, however, is that toxins—to which we are exposed from the air we breathe, the food and water we eat and drink, and even some of the cosmetic products we use—enter our bloodstreams and circulate throughout our bodies every day. Over time, they can build up in our systems, resulting in headaches, fatigue, muscle pain, indigestion, constipation, and a variety of other symptoms. And because these symptoms are fairly common and general, an accumulation of unwanted compounds in the bloodstream may not be the first cause that comes to mind when looking for solutions.

What's in Your Blood & Why You Should Care tells you everything you need to know about your blood and your body's natural detoxification mechanisms. It also reveals evidence-based methods of cleansing your bloodstream that you can incorporate into your normal daily routine. With a wealth of information on diets to supplements to complementary therapies, this book is designed to show you a pathway to better health.

This book is divided into three parts. Part One begins by detailing the composition of your blood, from plasma and red blood cells to white blood cells and platelets. It then discusses the ways in which your pH balance, diet, level of physical activity, environment, and genetics influence the state of your blood. It also provides a chapter all about blood tests, listing each element and describing what it can tell you about the status of your health. Finally, it explains how toxins may enter your bloodstream due to external exposure or internal biological processes, and outlines how your body's natural detoxification mechanisms go about eliminating these substances from your body.

Part Two talks about the six types of nutrients that your body requires for proper health—carbohydrates, fat, protein, vitamins, minerals, and water—and how they work together in the production of energy, the promotion of cell growth, and the achievement of proper organ function once they have been absorbed into your bloodstream. It goes on to discuss how the foods you choose to eat each day can have an enormous impact on your blood and thus on your health. It then describes the importance of optimal oxygen levels in your blood, why your blood may be depleted of oxygen, and how to increase oxygen levels in your blood.

Part Three ties everything together by detailing particular foods and supplements that encourage detoxification of your blood, as well as the benefits of occasional fasting. It concludes by recommending complementary therapies that may be used to promote the detoxification process and help you maintain a healthy bloodstream, including sauna therapy, hydrotherapy, massage therapy, chelation therapy, and meditation.

When it comes to your health and well-being, you may feel as though you are a helpless bystander, simply waiting to see all the cards in the hand you have been dealt genetically. While genetics, no doubt, play a powerful role in your health, you can play an active part as well. Through the choices you make every day, you can prevent harmful substances from entering your bloodstream in the first place and support the elimination of unwanted compounds in your circulatory system.

PART ONE

What You Need to Know About Your Blood

Part One of this book is designed to provide you with a basic understanding of the components of your blood, how your blood works in your body, what a blood test reveals, and the ways in which your body's natural detoxification mechanisms eliminate unwanted substances from your bloodstream. Chapter 1 discusses the composition of your blood, factors that affect it, and how your blood travels throughout your body. Chapter 2 lists the various measurements of a traditional blood test and explains how the results of these measurements can offer you a picture of your health status. Finally, Chapter 3 defines external and internal toxins, notes how these compounds may enter your bloodstream, and details how your body's natural detoxification mechanisms go about eliminating these substances from your body.

1

All About Your Blood

Blood is the primary means of transport for both the helpful and the harmful substances inside your body. This vital fluid carries such things as vitamins, minerals, oxygen, hormones, heavy metals, and even toxins through your cellular pathways. These chemical compounds reach your blood once they have been taken in by your body, whether deliberately or unintentionally, from the environment, and then get distributed throughout your system as your blood circulates.

Your circulatory system contains about 1.3 gallons, or 5 liters, of blood at any given time, which comes into contact with virtually all the trillions of cells in your body. Given its expansive role, blood could be considered the common denominator of your well-being. This chapter explains the composition of blood, factors that affect it, blood types, and how blood travels throughout your body.

THE COMPOSITION OF BLOOD

The circulatory system has been compared to the canals of Venice. Just as this Italian city's waterways allow travelers to go from one place to another, your blood picks up and drops off "passengers" throughout your body on a continuous basis. Your arteries, veins, and capillaries are, in essence, a vast network of "canals"—so vast, in fact, that if you lined up all the veins, arteries, and capillaries found in the average person, they would wrap around the world twice! But just as Venice's canals are used by a variety of boats that take people and cargo from location to location, your blood comprises many different working parts. Each of these parts serves the same important purpose, which is to sustain human life. To better understand how your blood performs this task, you must first learn about its primary components, which include plasma, red blood cells, white blood cells, and platelets.[1]

■ PLASMA

Plasma is a yellow liquid that holds blood cells in suspension. About 55 percent of your blood is plasma, and about 92 percent of plasma is water. Most of the remaining 8 percent of plasma is made up of proteins, while small amounts of glucose, clotting factors, electrolytes, hormones, and carbon dioxide make up the remainder.

Water

Given that plasma is primarily water—and given that the human body is made up of about 55- to 65-percent water—it is helpful to understand the role water serves in the body. To begin with, water is the fluid that allows plasma (and all components of blood) to circulate freely throughout your body. Without adequate water, plasma would be sludge in your veins, arteries, and capillaries. In addition, plasma, which acts as the major delivery system for water, transports water to the parts of your body that need it, moistening your tissues (e.g., mouth, eyes, and nose), lubricating your joints, protecting your organs and tissues by preventing their dehydration, helping to dissolve minerals and other nutrients to make them biologically accessible, regulating your body temperature, and flushing waste products from your kidneys and liver. Almost all major systems of your body depend on water, which is why you're always hearing about the importance of drinking enough fluids.

Plasma Proteins

The word "protein" is derived from the Greek word "proteios," which essentially means "of primary importance." Indeed, after water, proteins are the most common substances in your body. But what exactly are they? *Proteins* are structures that help your body execute a wide variety of functions, including moving molecules from one place to another, replicating DNA, and cell signaling, which refers to the way in which cells communicate with each other.

Proteins are composed of various combinations of *amino acids,* which act as their building blocks. Some amino acids come from the protein in the foods you eat, while others are produced by your body. Animal-derived food sources of protein include beef, poultry, dairy, and seafood. Vegetarian sources of protein include seeds, nuts, legumes (beans, lentils, peanuts, etc.).

During digestion, the proteins in your food are typically broken down by your intestines into their component amino acids, which are then absorbed into your bloodstream. Sometimes, however, a protein isn't completely broken down into amino acids but rather into partial proteins, or small amino-acid chains. A partial protein is known as a *peptide* and is categorized according to its number of amino acids. For example, a *tripeptide* has three amino acids, while a *dipeptide* has two amino acids. Small peptides may be absorbed into your bloodstream.

Amino acids can join together to create many different proteins, including specialized proteins found in muscles, hormones, and even plasma itself. In fact, proteins are the second most prevalent substance in plasma. The protein *albumin* accounts for about 55 percent of the various proteins in plasma. *Globulin* makes up about 38 percent. *Fibrinogen* makes up about 7 percent. These proteins perform a great number of vital tasks, including the transport of hormones, fats, vitamins, and minerals throughout your circulatory system, as well as the functioning of your immune system.

In fact, *antibodies,* which account for a significant portion of a type of globulin called *gamma globulin,* are large Y-shaped proteins produced predominantly by plasma cells as part of your body's overall immune response. Also known as *immunoglobulins,* they are used to neutralize disease-causing microorganisms, also known as *pathogens,* such as bacteria and viruses. The two tips of an antibody's Y shape fit a certain *antigen,* which is a unique molecule residing on the surface of a pathogen, like a lock and key. When an antibody recognizes its corresponding antigen, it binds to it. This action can neutralize the antigen directly or call on other parts of your immune system to destroy the molecule. Different antibodies are specific to different antigens.

■ RED BLOOD CELLS

Red blood cells (RBCs), also called *erythrocytes,* are disc-shaped cells that are concave on both sides. Their job is to transport oxygen throughout your body while also bringing carbon dioxide to your lungs for you to exhale. RBCs make up nearly 40 to 45 percent of your blood's volume. They are produced in your bone marrow, starting out as immature stem cells, which can mature into virtually any type of cell required by your body. This process takes about seven days, after which the new RBCs are released into your bloodstream through your bones. Once in your blood, red blood cells have an average life span of 120 days.

When your RBCs have recently taken oxygen from your lungs, the color of your blood is bright red. After releasing oxygen into your body's tissues, the color is more of a dark red. It is, in fact, the hemoglobin found within red blood cells that provides the red color of blood.

Hemoglobin

Hemoglobin is a red iron-containing protein in red blood cells that binds to oxygen, allowing its transport throughout your body.

Hemoglobin is also involved in returning carbon dioxide (the waste product of oxygen) from your tissues back to your lungs.[2] Hemoglobin also plays an important role in maintaining the shape of red blood cells. An abnormal hemoglobin structure (e.g., the sickle-like shape of hemoglobin found in sickle cell anemia) can disrupt the shape of red blood cells and impede their function and movement through blood vessels.

RBC Antigens

Normally, an antigen is a substance on a pathogen, such as a bacteria or a virus, whose very presence stimulates your immune system into action, attracting specific antibodies floating in your plasma to neutralize that antigen. As it turns out, however, each red blood cell is also covered with antigens composed of either sugar or protein. The purpose of most of these *RBC antigens* is unknown and, in most cases, they are ignored by your immune system. There are two specific types of RBC antigens, though, that are different from the others. They have been identified as *A antigens* and *B antigens*. If you have A antigens on your RBCs, then your plasma will also contain *B antibodies*, which will mobilize a targeted immune response when exposed to B antigens from foreign blood. Similarly, if you have B antigens, then your plasma's *A antibodies* will attack any A antigens from outside blood sources. The discovery of these antigens and their effects led to the important classification of blood according to blood type. (See "Antigens and Blood Type" on page 10.)

While the purpose of RBC antigens remains unknown, it is nevertheless clear that they set off antibody responses when they come into contact with any red blood cells that are incompatible. If a person with a given blood type receives a transfusion of blood of the same blood type, then that person's plasma antibodies will not react and his or her immune system will recognize the incoming antigens as "friends" rather than "foes." If, on the other hand, a person receives a blood type that is not his or her own, then the antibodies in that person's plasma will attack and his

ANTIGENS AND BLOOD TYPE

In the early 1800s, doctors began to transfuse blood from one person to another in hopes of replacing a patient's lost blood. Unfortunately, deadly consequences followed in many cases. It was not until 1900 that Austrian scientist Karl Landsteiner discovered the cause of such reactions: conflicting blood types. It was found that each person has a particular blood type based on the RBC antigens inherited from his or her parents, and that a transfusion of a different blood type to one's own could be deadly.

To explain, if you inherit the A antigen, then you will be blood type A and your plasma will have B antibodies. If you inherit the B antigen, then you will be blood type B and your plasma will contain A antibodies. If you inherit both antigens, then you will be blood type AB and your plasma will contain neither A nor B antibodies. And if you do not inherit either the A or B antigen, leaving the surface of your RBCs "blank," then you will be blood type O and your plasma will contain both A and B antibodies. In addition to this letter-based classification, if you inherit what is known as the *Rh factor* antigen, then your blood will be *Rh positive*. If you do not, then your blood will be *Rh negative*. This is typically written as a plus [+] or minus [–] after your ABO blood type (e.g., A+, O–). In total, the presence or absence of these antigens accounts for eight different blood types: A+, A–, B+, B–, AB+, AB–, O+, and O–.

Some blood types are common and others are rare. Table 1.1 on the following page shows the prevalence of each blood type in the United States according to ethnic group.

or her immune system will reject the transfused blood—seeing its antigens as foreign invaders. This reaction can lead to a catastrophic result. Successful blood transfusions depend on careful blood typing and cross-matching. In short, the presence or absence of specific antigens on the surface of a patient's red blood cells dictates which blood types that patient may safely receive from a blood donor. (See Table 1.2 on page 11.)

TABLE 1.1. COMMON BLOOD TYPES IN THE UNITED STATES BY ETHNIC GROUP			
	Caucasians	**African-American**	**Hispanic**	**Asian**
O+	37 percent	47 percent	53 percent	39 percent
O–	8 percent	4 percent	4 percent	1 percent
A+	33 percent	24 percent	29 percent	27 percent
A–	7 percent	2 percent	2 percent	0.5 percent
B+	9 percent	18 percent	9 percent	25 percent
B–	2 percent	1 percent	1 percent	0.4 percent
AB+	3 percent	4 percent	2 percent	7 percent
AB–	1 percent	0.3 percent	0.2 percent	0.1 percent

In terms of RBCs, blood type O is what is known as the *universal donor*. It can donate blood to anybody. Blood type AB can donate only to others of the AB type (although it is the universal donor of plasma). Moreover, blood type AB is the *universal recipient*, being able to receive RBCs from any blood type. This rule is mitigated, however, by the presence or absence of the Rh factor. For the most part, Rh-negative blood is given to Rh-negative patients, and Rh-positive blood or Rh-negative blood may be given to Rh-positive patients.

TABLE 1.2. BLOOD DONOR GUIDE			
Patient's Blood Type	**Antigen on surface of RBC**	**Antibody in Plasma**	**Donor Blood Type**
A	A antigen	B antibody	A, O
B	B antigen	A antibody	B, O
AB	Both A and B antigens	Neither A nor B antibody	A, B, AB, O
O	Neither A nor B	A and B antibody	O

◼ WHITE BLOOD CELLS

White blood cells (WBCs), also referred to as *leukocytes*, make up 2 percent of your blood and are a marker of the health of your immune system. There are five general types of WBCs, which protect your body from bacteria and other harmful substances.[3,4] As with red blood cells, WBCs start as immature stem cells in your bone marrow. Once released into your bloodstream, white blood cells have a lifespan that ranges from thirteen to twenty days. The five different types of WBCs—neutrophils, eosinophils, basophils, lymphocytes, and monocytes—perform different roles in your immune system.

Neutrophils

Neutrophils are the most abundant type of white blood cell in your body, making up about 62 percent of WBCs. They are "first responders" to the presence of inflammation, especially inflammation caused by the presence of bacteria. Their main targets are bacteria and fungi.

Eosinophils

Eosinophils make up about 2.3 percent of WBCs. They are one of your immune system's main components for combating multicellular parasites and certain infections, while some eosinophils also play a role in fighting viral infections. In addition, they help control mechanisms associated with allergies and asthma.

Basophils

Basophils make up about 0.4 percent of WBCs. They are responsible for many inflammatory reactions and can perform phagocytosis, which refers to the ingestion of certain foreign invaders, such as bacteria, by specific cells. Basophils also produce *histamine* and *serotonin,* which induce inflammation, and play a role in preventing blood clotting.

Lymphocytes

Lymphocytes make up about 30 percent of WBCs. Lymphocytes can be divided into three types: *B cells, natural killer cells,* and *T cells.* B cells are involved mainly in the release of antibodies and the activation of T cells. Natural killer cells predominantly attack virus-infected cells and tumor cells. T cells are further divided into four subtypes: *T helper cells, cytotoxic T cells, gamma delta T cells,* and *regulatory T cells.* T helper cells activate and regulate T and B cells. Cytotoxic T cells go after virus-infected and tumor cells. Gamma delta T cells function as a bridge between innate immunity (the early phase of your immune system's response to infection) and adaptive immunity (the formation of immune chemicals—e.g., antibodies—designed for specific foreign invaders). Finally, regulatory T cells return the state of your immune system to normal after an infection and also help prevent auto-immune responses.

Monocytes

Monocytes make up about 5.3 percent of WBCs and are the largest type of white blood cell. They migrate from the bloodstream to other tissues, becoming resident *macrophages,* which are a specialized type of WBC that engulfs and digests cellular debris, foreign substances, microbes, and cancer cells.

■ PLATELETS

Platelets, also referred to as *thrombocytes,* are fragments of *cytoplasm* (i.e., material living within a cell, excluding the nucleus) derived from cells of bone marrow. They are tiny in size—only about 20-percent of the size of a red blood cell—and represent a small fraction of your blood. Despite their tiny size, they perform a crucial function. Specifically, they help blood clump and clot around the site of a blood vessel injury, plugging the hole (unless it is too large).[5]

The State of Your Blood

A combination of plasma, red blood cells, white blood cells, and platelets forms your blood. These individual components perform important functions necessary for your health and well-being. Of course, the state of your blood can be altered by a number of influences. If you recognize these many influences, you can try to make the appropriate changes to your lifestyle that can help you keep your blood healthy.

WHAT INFLUENCES THE STATE OF YOUR BLOOD?

Now that you have a basic understanding of the components that make up your blood, let's take a look at five critical factors—pH balance, diet, physical activity, environment, and genetics—that influence the state of your blood.

pH Balance

The *pH scale* is a measure of how *acidic* or *alkaline* (also known as *basic*) a substance is. The scale ranges from 0 to 14—with a pH number of 7 considered neutral, a pH number less than 7 considered acidic, and a pH number greater than 7 considered alkaline. An important concept in pH is that each whole pH value below 7 is ten times more acidic than the next higher value, and a pH value above 7 is ten times more alkaline. For example, a pH reading of 4 is ten times more acidic than a pH reading of 5, and 100 times more acidic than a pH reading of 6. Consequently, even small changes in pH can be significant.

The pH of your blood is tightly controlled by your body, which works to keep your pH level from being too acidic or too basic. Your body achieves this balance by introducing natural substances into your blood, including carbonic acid, bicarbonate, and carbon dioxide—all substances that your body already has in residence.[6,7] It should be noted, however, that the contemporary North American diet tends to be high in animal protein and relatively low in fruit and vegetables. This manner of eating can cause an acidic pH in an otherwise healthy adult subject.

When your body becomes too acidic, proteins can start to break down, *enzymes* (molecules that act as biological catalysts, accelerating chemical reactions in your body) can begin to lose their ability to function, and other negative effects may occur. For example, research suggests that acidity may be associated with the development of ovarian cancer and possibly other cancers as well.[8] Other research indicates that an acidic pH may contribute to the development of mucous membrane injury on the lining of the esophagus in connection with gastroesophageal reflux disease, or GERD.[9] In addition, research has identified that acidity promotes mineral loss in bones.[10,11,12,13]

Diet

A healthy diet, or lack thereof, has a profound effect on the health of all cells, tissues, organs, and bodily systems—your blood is no exception. In fact, the very production of red blood cells in your body is dependent upon the availability of key vitamins and minerals derived from your diet. These vitamins and minerals include the following:

- **Copper.** Alongside iron, the chemical element *copper* is a necessary component in the formation of red blood cells.

- **Folic Acid.** *Folic acid* is necessary in the formation of both red blood cells and white blood cells.

- **Iron.** *Iron* is a chemical element and the part of the hemoglobin protein used to carry oxygen throughout your body. Without sufficient iron, the result would be *anemia,* which is a health condition characterized by an insufficient production of red blood cells.

- **Vitamin B$_{12}$.** *Vitamin B$_{12}$* is required in the formation of red blood cells in bone marrow. A shortage of B$_{12}$ can cause a type of anemia called pernicious anemia.

- **Vitamin C.** *Vitamin C* helps in the absorption of iron. A shortage can lead to a small-cell-type anemia known as microcytic anemia.

Certain dietary vitamins (including vitamins C, E, and A) also serve as *antioxidants,* which help prevent free radicals from harming your cells and cardiovascular system. *Free radicals* are essentially chemical "buzz bombs" that damage cellular structures, including DNA. A diet lacking in sufficient fruits and vegetables means that you won't be getting much in the way of antioxidant protection from your food. Unfortunately, research from the United States Department of Agriculture (USDA) has shown that Americans are consuming about 50-percent less fruit and 40-percent less vegetables than we should be.[14] In fact, the USDA has indicated that only 10 percent of Americans actually eat what might be considered a good diet.[15,16]

Diet also affects your blood indirectly through its effect on your pH level, which, as previously explained, influences the state of your blood. Research suggests that human beings would be better off following a similar diet to that of our ancestors rather than the one we have adopted since the agricultural revolution (10,000 years ago) and industrialization (200 years ago).[17]

Specifically, a critical difference between our ancestors' diet and our current diet is that we eat far less potassium-rich foods (present in the plant foods that our ancestors ate in abundance).

Rather, we now have an over-abundance of sodium chloride (salt) in our contemporary diet, and a relatively meager intake of potassium-rich plant foods. In fact, other research suggests that the ratio of our potassium to sodium intake has reversed from a previous 10:1 to 1:3 thanks to our modern eating habits.[18] The bottom line is that this ratio reversal, with its deficiency of potassium intake, increases the likelihood of a more acidic system, which negatively affects your blood.

Physical Activity

Physical activity has a profound effect on your blood and cardiovascular system. It is well established that exercise promotes healthy circulation, which, of course, is needed to move blood throughout your body at an effective rate. Only one in five Americans, however, meets the Physical Activity Guidelines for Americans, which recommend getting at least two and half hours of physical activity each week (30 minutes of exercise five days per week).[19] As a result, as many as 250,000 deaths every year in the United States may be attributable to a lack of regular physical activity.[20]

Although there are many benefits associated with exercise, those specific to blood and cardiovascular health include lowering your blood pressure, reducing "bad cholesterol" (low-density lipoprotein, or LDL, cholesterol) in your blood, lowering your total cholesterol, and raising your "good cholesterol" (high-density lipoprotein, or HDL, cholesterol) levels. In addition, exercise improves your body's ability to take in and use oxygen (known as *maximal oxygen consumption*). As this ability improves, your regular daily activities may be performed with less fatigue. There is also evidence that exercise training enhances the capacity of your blood vessels to dilate in response to exercise or hormones, which is associated with improved functioning of blood vessel walls.[21]

Environment

In her groundbreaking 1962 book *Silent Spring*, Rachel Carson writes, "For the first time in the history of the world every human being is now subjected to contact with dangerous chemicals, from the moment of conception until death." Of course, humans have always been exposed to potentially harmful chemicals from plants and other sources, but Rachel Carson's point is well taken. Modern living exposes all of us to an unprecedented number of chemicals on a daily basis, including environmental toxins such as heavy metals, pesticides, industrial compounds and byproducts, medications, cosmetic additives, and inorganic chemicals. In fact, according to the Environmental Protection Agency (EPA), in 2010, about 3.97 billion pounds of toxic chemicals were disposed of or otherwise released into the environment.[22]

This toxic exposure can have an adverse effect on the health of your blood and your organ systems in general—regardless of your profession, education, age, or sex.[23] In fact, chronic exposure to environmental toxins may result in headache, fatigue, poor memory, inflammation, pain, or gastrointestinal discomfort.[24,25] Moreover, while environmental toxins can affect the health of your blood, it is your blood that carries these toxins throughout your body, delivering them to some of the areas where they can cause the greatest harm.

Genetics

Heredity—the many traits you inherit from your parents—can play a profound role in the health and functioning of your body, including your blood. Genetics is the study of heredity and inherited characteristics.

You've probably seen pictures of the double-helix referred to as DNA, which functions as the genetic "blueprint" that provides all the information necessary to make a human being. DNA is made up of individual *genes*, which are grouped into *chromosomes*.

GENETIC BLOOD DISORDERS

Genetic blood disorders include those that are passed down through families and affect the normal properties of blood in humans. Their effects can range from benign to lethal. The following is a brief discussion of the most common genetic blood disorders.

• **Hemochromatosis.** This term refers to the accumulation of too much iron in the body, which can be caused by a genetic disorder. Symptoms may include cirrhosis of the liver, diabetes, cardiomyopathy, joint and bone pain, testicular failure, and bronzing of the skin. Treatment generally consists of drawing blood until iron levels are brought into normal range.[27]

• **Hemophilia.** This bleeding disorder is caused by a genetic lack of blood clotting factor. The result can be bleeding for a greater length of time than normal after an injury, bruising easily, and an increased risk of bleeding inside joints or the brain.[28]

• **Porphyria.** This disorder affects the way that *heme* (the red pigment in hemoglobin) is made. The resulting symptoms may include abdominal pain, chest pain, vomiting, confusion, constipation, fever, and seizures.[29]

• **Sickle cell anemia.** This well-known genetic blood disorder is characterized by an abnormality in the hemoglobin that results in a rigid, sickle-like shape to RBCs rather than the typical disc shape. Sickle cell anemia can lead to attacks of pain, bacterial infections, and stroke, as well as long-term pain as the affected individual gets older.[30]

• **Thalassemia.** This genetic blood disorder is characterized by abnormally formed hemoglobin. It often leads to a low RBC count (i.e., anemia), which, in turn, can result in fatigue, pale skin, and several other symptoms, although sometimes it leads to no symptoms at all.[31]

In addition to these inherited blood disorders, there are genetic influences in certain disease states. One such example is *leukemia*, a group of different cancers of the blood in which bone marrow and other blood-forming organs produce increased numbers of immature or abnormal leukocytes, or white blood cells. These leukocytes suppress the production of normal blood cells, leading to anemia and other symptoms. Some people have a genetic predisposition towards developing leukemia. In some cases, families tend to develop the same kind of leukemia; in other families, those affected may develop different forms of the disease.[32]

Human beings have forty-six chromosomes—twenty-three are inherited from each parent. These genes provide instructions for manufacturing the proteins that make up the human body. If there is a genetic error in one or more genes, this can result in the wrong protein being made, which, in turn, can result in a greater likelihood of disease development or other problems. When we think of heredity and blood, the first thing that generally comes to mind is blood type. (See page 10.) But blood type is neither good nor bad in regard to health. There are certain genetic blood disorders, however, which can interfere with the way your blood does its job and, consequently, with your health. While the genetic factors involved in disease seem to be out of your control, since you obviously cannot change the genes you inherited, the good news is that, in some cases, you can exert some influence on how your genes perform, which may have a desirable impact on certain disease processes.[26] This concept is known as epigenetics.

Epigenetics

Your genes are not just a blueprint of genetic material for reproducing cells. Each day they are actively involved in producing certain proteins that perform various functions in your body. Moreover, the nutrients and other natural compounds you acquire from the foods you eat can actually affect gene expression, flipping genetic "switches" on or off, and changing how certain proteins are made. The study of the modification of gene expression is known as *epigenetics,* and such alterations can be crucial in relation to the genes that play a role in facilitating or preventing the disease process.

Since your blood carries these epigenetically important substances to your cells, and ultimately to your genes, the health of your blood, coupled with an effectively functioning cardiovascular system, is critical in ensuring that your genes express themselves in ways that prevent disease and not encourage it.[33]

THE BLOOD VESSELS

To better understand of the way in which your blood circulates throughout your body, let us first take a look at the types of "canals" through which your blood speeds to complete its cardiovascular journey: arteries, veins, and capillaries.

Arteries are blood vessels that carry your blood away from your heart, at which point your blood branches into ever-smaller vessels. With the exception of your *pulmonary artery*, which carries deoxygenated blood from your heart to your lungs, and the *umbilical arteries*, which supply a pregnant woman's placenta with deoxygenated blood from her fetus, your arteries carry oxygenated blood to sustain the rest of your body. They are thicker than your veins, as they are closer to your heart and receive blood surging forth at a much greater pressure. The hollow passageway through which blood flows within your arteries is also smaller than that of your veins, a trait which helps maintain the pressure of your blood as it is transported throughout your body. Unlike your veins, your arteries also have an inner muscular layer called the intima, which helps move blood along by way of smaller contractions.[34]

Veins are blood vessels that carry deoxygenated blood (blood that has already delivered its oxygen) to your heart, with the exception of your *pulmonary veins*, which move oxygenated blood to your heart, and the *umbilical vein*, which carries oxygenated blood from a pregnant woman's placenta to her growing fetus. Your veins are thinner than your arteries and have larger hollow passageways through which your blood flows. They lack the muscular layer that arteries have, but they are equipped with valves that allow your blood to keep moving forward and prevent its backflow. Your veins also deliver cellular wastes to your liver for processing.[35]

Capillaries are the smallest of blood vessels. In fact, the diameter of the hollow passageway in some capillaries is so small that there is just enough space to allow red blood cells to fit through one at a time. By virtue of being leaky, capillary walls allow the passage of oxygen, nutrients, and other critical substances to pass through to your cells. Conversely, toxins and waste materials can pass from your cells into your capillaries, where they can then travel to your veins and ultimately be metabolized and excreted from your body.[36]

THE PATHWAYS OF THE BLOOD

While in the womb, a baby doesn't need to use its own lungs because it receives oxygenated blood through its mother's placenta. Once a baby is born, however, that first breath of fresh oxygen allows its lungs to do the work of oxygenating its blood themselves. While the circulatory system moves blood through your body in a continuous loop, for all practical purposes, the lungs may be considered the start of the route taken by the blood—whether in a newborn or in an adult, it all starts in the lungs. In fact, in order to accurately visualize the path your blood takes, it is helpful to divide your overall cardiovascular system into two specific circuits: *pulmonary circulation* and *systemic circulation.*

Your heart has four separate chambers. The two largest are known as the *left ventricle* and the *right ventricle.* Pulmonary circulation refers to the movement of the blood in your heart's right ventricle (deoxygenated blood that has been brought to your heart from the rest of your body) into your lungs via your pulmonary artery, where it is then oxygenated, leaving behind carbon dioxide to be exhaled. It is important to note that the lungs of people who smoke or who are exposed to second-hand smoke may become damaged, making them less efficient at transferring oxygen and carbon dioxide to and from the bloodstream, respectively, while also substantially increasing their risk of lung cancer.[37] This oxygenated blood is then returned to your heart via your pulmonary veins, although this time it is deposited into your heart's left ventricle. Pulmonary circulation is the circuit that maintains the process of blood oxygenation and carbon dioxide expulsion. As your body relies on oxygenated blood to survive, this subtype of circulation is a vital component of the overall cardiovascular system.

Once oxygenated blood has been transferred to your heart's left ventricle, it is then ready for systemic circulation, which pumps the oxygen-rich blood away from your heart through its largest artery, the aorta, to the rest of your body with the exception of your lungs. The blood branches off into smaller and smaller arteries,

BLOOD FILTRATION

Systemic circulation includes a vessel called the *hepatic portal vein*, which actually carries blood and its nutrients from your gastrointestinal tract, spleen, gallbladder, and pancreas to capillaries in your liver before returning it to the heart. Your liver then directs each nutrient to its appropriate destination, sometimes storing certain of them to meet future needs, while filtering out any toxins that may have also come along. As such, your liver has a strong influence on the quality of your blood and your overall health. In its role as a filter, it allows many of the harmful substances found in your blood to hitch a ride out of your body on a greenish-brown fluid known as *bile*.

Bile is secreted by your liver to aid in fat digestion. It moves from your liver to your gallbladder to your intestines, at which point it is excreted in your fecal matter. In yet another example of the ingenious nature of the human body, the waste products filtered by your liver make their way out of your system by taking advantage of the pathway already used by bile. Understandably, it is critically important that the liver function at its very best for this detoxification process to occur properly.[38]

In addition, during systemic circulation, blood flows through your kidneys, two bean-shaped organs that also serve a blood-filtering role. These organs filter your blood to produce *urine*, which contains certain substances that have been filtered out by your kidneys. Urine is released into your bladder through a tube known as the *ureter* and then exits your body through a tube known as the *urethra*. In general, your kidneys filter out smaller, water-soluble waste matter, while your liver filters out larger, fat-soluble compounds.[39]

and finally into the capillaries in your tissues. Your capillaries then make the necessary exchange of chemical compounds with your tissues at the cellular level, leaving behind oxygen, glucose, and nutrients while taking carbon dioxide and other metabolic waste. Once this exchange has been made, veins carry the deoxygenated blood back to the heart, where the whole process begins again. This propulsion of blood can be felt with each beat of your heart. Your heart beats about 108,000 times each day, or 39 million times per year.

CONCLUSION

A well-functioning cardiovascular system is crucial to the proper flow of blood throughout your body, which is designed to deliver gases and nutrients to your cells, and to take waste material away from your cells. With the help of organs such as your liver and kidneys, these problematic substances may then be filtered from your blood and expelled from your body. While this chapter may be a simplified look at the cardiovascular system, it encompasses the essence of how blood keeps each of us alive and functioning. The individual components of your blood, the vessels and organs involved in your circulatory system, and the way in which they all work together make for a truly remarkable mechanism. And as you will come to understand in the chapters that follow, the more you know about this ever-flowing river of life, the more control you will have over your well-being.

2

What Your Blood Test Reveals

No book about what's in your blood would be complete without a chapter on blood tests—what they are and what they can tell you about your health status. In general, blood tests are performed to check for disorders, dysfunction, and disease on the basis of whether the substances being measured in your blood fall into a normal or abnormal range. Furthermore, a blood test is one of the best ways to ensure that your diet, lifestyle, and medication (if you are already being treated for a particular condition) are doing their jobs. The bottom line is that a blood test is a good way to measure the state of your health and allow you to manage it more effectively and easily.

This chapter has been organized into six sections. The first four sections focus on the four traditional blood panels (specific groupings of blood tests), which include the lipid panel, the basic metabolic panel, the hepatic function panel, and the complete blood count (CBC). The fifth section looks at commonly administered hormone tests, while the sixth section reviews additional tests that, although not routinely administered, provide a more complete picture of your well-being.[1]

■ THE LIPID PANEL YOUR FAT LEVELS AND HEART HEALTH

The *lipid panel* consists of blood tests used to evaluate your heart health. This panel includes four types of measurement of the fat found in your blood: triglycerides, total cholesterol, high-density lipoprotein (HDL), and low-density lipoprotein (LDL). Homocysteine and C-reactive protein (CRP) levels provide two additional measurements of cardiovascular health, although descriptions of these readings are included in the section on optional tests. (See page 43.)

BLOOD TEST ACCURACY

Depending upon a number of lifestyle factors, a standard blood test may or may not always be completely accurate. These factors include your intake of certain foods, physical activity levels, alcohol consumption habits, daily caffeine intake, and use of certain medications. Any of these aspects of your everyday life may influence the results of your blood test, which is why it is so important to follow the instructions given to you by your doctor before you have your blood drawn. If you're told to fast for a certain number of hours before having your blood taken, make sure to do so, otherwise you risk abnormal findings on your blood test, which may lead to false positive or false negative results.

Triglycerides

Triglycerides make up the primary form of *fat*, or *lipid*, in your blood. They perform an important role, serving as a source of fuel for your body's energy production. The majority of the fats you eat, whether healthy or unhealthy ones, fall under the category of triglycerides. While your body requires a certain amount of fat to remain healthy, overly elevated levels can lead to health problems such as heart disease. Simply put, if you consume unnecessarily large amounts of food, your body will be left with unused calories, which it will convert into triglycerides to be stored in fat cells, making you fatter. In addition, an excess of triglycerides circulating throughout your bloodstream (known as *hypertriglyceridemia*) is a major risk factor for heart disease, diabetes, insulin resistance, metabolic syndrome, and liver disease. The reason that excess triglycerides represent such a risk is that they can combine with cholesterol to form other fatty molecules such as very low-density lipoprotein (VLDL), which, in turn, may contribute to the formation of arterial plaque and promote inflammation.

When you push your body to burn more energy, however, such as through exercise, certain hormones are then produced that can signal the release of triglycerides from fat cells so that they may be burned as fuel, resulting in weight loss. Although the fat content of your diet is an important consideration when it comes to your health, you must also be careful of eating foods that contain a lot of sugar or refined carbohydrates, which are easily converted into triglycerides and often lead to weight gain, contributing to heart disease and other health problems.

Total Cholesterol

Despite negative press it has received, *cholesterol* actually plays an important role in the health of your body. Produced by your liver, this fat is required to create cell membranes. It is also necessary to produce bile for fat digestion and serves as the principal building block of many hormones (including estrogen, testosterone, and progesterone) and vitamin D. In addition to your liver's production of cholesterol, dietary sources of cholesterol also contribute to the levels found in your bloodstream. These sources include beef, dairy products, and eggs.

Lipoprotein contains cholesterol, triglycerides, and protein. Essentially, your total cholesterol reading is the sum of your *high-density lipoprotein* (HDL), *low-density lipoprotein* (LDL), and *very low-density lipoprotein* (VLDL) levels. HDL cholesterol is often referred to as "good" cholesterol, as it carries cholesterol away from your arteries to your liver, where it can be removed from your body. LDL cholesterol is generally considered "bad" cholesterol, as it delivers cholesterol through your bloodstream, which can contribute to your risk of clogged arteries. Very low-density lipoprotein (VLDL) contains the highest amount of triglycerides of the three lipoproteins in question, but because there is no direct way to measure VLDL, it is not typically mentioned when your doctor assesses your blood work. Another important factor in determining cholesterol's total effect on your body is the particle size of cholesterol. Larger HDL particles are more beneficial than smaller HDL particles. Likewise, the more oxidized (i.e., damaged) LDL particles present, the more likely the development of plaque buildup and *atherosclerosis*, which refers to the hardening and narrowing of your arteries. People with "borderline high" or "high" total cholesterol levels are at higher risk of heart disease than those with normal readings.

Low-Density Lipoprotein (LDL) Cholesterol

LDL cholesterol transports about 70 percent of the cholesterol in your body through your bloodstream to your cells and tissues. When LDL is oxidized it becomes even more harmful than regular LDL, contributing to artery blockage, thereby setting the stage for heart disease and *peripheral artery disease*, which refers to the narrowing of your peripheral arteries (most commonly of the arteries to your legs). In turn, these conditions can lead to heart attack, stroke, or blood clots. Without a doubt, high LDL levels are a dangerous and potentially fatal problem. In fact, the target range for LDL values has dropped progressively over the last decade as scientists have learned more about this substance and the health dangers it poses.

High-Density Lipoprotein (HDL) Cholesterol

HDL cholesterol is referred to as "good" cholesterol because it carries "bad" cholesterol to your liver, where it is then removed from your system. Consequently, it is actually desirable to have an elevated level of HDL. Basically, HDL performs the job of a cleaning crew that locates and cleans out the cholesterol that causes clogged arteries. Maintaining a favorable level of HDL significantly reduces the risk of *coronary artery disease.*

■ THE BASIC METABOLIC PANEL
YOUR SUGAR LEVELS, ELECTROLYE BALANCE & KIDNEY HEALTH

The *basic metabolic panel* evaluates blood sugar regulation, electrolyte and fluid balance, and kidney function. The *biomarkers* (short for "biological markers," which refer to quantifiable indicators of certain biological states) measured in this panel include glucose, calcium, potassium, sodium, chloride, carbon dioxide, blood urea nitrogen (BUN), and creatinine.

Glucose

Glucose, or *blood sugar*, acts as your body's primary source of energy. Carbohydrates found in food, including sugars and starches, are ultimately broken down into three simple sugars: *fructose, galactose,* and *glucose.* Fructose and galactose may be further converted into glucose and used as fuel. When your glucose levels rise, your pancreas releases *insulin,* a hormone that allows glucose to be taken out of your blood, carried to your cells, and used in energy production. But an excessive intake of carbohydrate-rich food and sugar can contribute to blood sugar imbalance. This may take the form of *high blood sugar,* or *hyperglycemia,* which can develop into *diabetes,* a condition in which your body can no longer produce or respond to insulin. In addition, *low blood sugar,* or *hypoglycemia,* may occur if too much insulin is released, triggering symptoms such as anxiousness, agitation, dizziness, sweating, and weakness. Poorly controlled blood sugar has been linked to Alzheimer's disease, Parkinson's disease, and autoimmune disorders.

Calcium

Calcium is the most plentiful mineral in the human body. The average healthy adult body contains between two and three pounds of this substance. Not only is calcium essential to the health of your bones and teeth, but it is also required for nerve impulse transmission, enzyme function, blood clotting, and energy production. It is known as an *electrolyte,* which is a substance that dissociates into ions when dissolved in a solvent. These ions create an electrically conductive solution in your system, which is required for muscle contraction and the stability of cell membranes.

Calcium levels are regulated by vitamin D, *parathyroid hormone* (PTH)—which increases blood calcium—and *calcitonin*—which decreases blood calcium. Magnesium and phosphorus levels in your body also affect your calcium levels.

Maintaining an adequate calcium intake is important. This may be achieved by eating calcium-rich foods, which include dairy products, fish that have bones (such as salmon and sardines), leafy green vegetables, and sesame seeds. Supplemental sources of calcium can also help. Insufficient intake of calcium over the long-term can lead to *osteoporosis,* which refers to the gradual thinning of bone tissue and loss of bone density.

Potassium

Potassium is also a mineral that functions as an electrolyte. It is necessary for proper nerve impulse transmission and muscle contraction, as well as crucial to other functions. This mineral helps maintain nerve and muscle growth, heart function, and a balanced pH level. It also assists in the cellular metabolism of carbohydrates and proteins. In addition, adequate potassium intake aids in lowering your blood pressure and thus your risk of stroke. If your potassium level becomes chronically low, you are also more likely to develop diabetes within the next decade of life.

Sodium

Like calcium and potassium, *sodium* is another mineral that functions as an electrolyte. It influences blood pressure regulation, heart rhythm, muscle contraction, and nerve impulse transmission. The current Dietary Guidelines for Americans recommend that Americans consume less than 2,300 milligrams (mg) of sodium each day as part of a healthy eating pattern.[2] The average daily sodium intake among individuals aged two years and older in the United States, however, is more than 3,400 mg per day—significantly higher than the recommended daily maximum.[3] This is highly problematic since, as sodium intake rises, so does blood pressure—and nearly sixty-eight million US adults (one in three) have high blood pressure.[4] If all Americans followed the recommended limits for sodium, national rates for high blood pressure would drop by one quarter, saving tens of thousands of lives each year.[5]

Chloride

Chloride, an electrolyte, is typically consumed in the form of sodium chloride, also known as table salt. In addition, chloride plays an important role in your metabolism while also helping your body maintain proper blood volume, blood pressure, and acid-alkaline balance (i.e., pH level). Typically, excess chloride is excreted in your urine. Abnormal chloride levels can reflect a problem with your kidneys, hormones, acid-alkaline balance, or electrolyte levels.

Carbon Dioxide

Carbon dioxide (CO_2) is one of the byproducts of *cellular respiration,* which refers to the process by which energy is produced by your body. When glucose, which contains carbon, is broken down in the presence of oxygen during cellular respiration, carbon dioxide is one result, along with water and, of course, energy. This carbon dioxide is taken up by your red blood cells and turned into *carbonic acid* (H_2CO_3). Most of this carbonic acid then becomes *bicarbonate* (HCO_3), which acts as an alkaline buffer in your blood, maintaining its pH balance. Most carbon dioxide in your blood (about 90 percent), in fact, takes the form of bicarbonate. Therefore, if your doctor orders a blood CO_2 test, the result will essentially reflect the amount of bicarbonate in your blood. Both high and low levels of carbon dioxide in your blood may indicate a pH or electrolyte imbalance.

Blood Urea Nitrogen (BUN)

Blood urea nitrogen (BUN) is a waste product of the digestion of protein. Your liver breaks down the proteins used by your cells, producing *ammonia,* which contains *nitrogen,* as a result. The nitrogen in this ammonia then combines with other elements to become *urea.* Urea is transported via your bloodstream to your kidneys, which filter this substance from your blood, allowing it to be eliminated from your body through your urine. As a result, kidney function should always be considered if your BUN levels are higher or lower than normal. In fact, reasons for a BUN test include suspected kidney dysfunction, heart or liver failure, urinary tract obstruction, and gastrointestinal bleeding.

Creatinine

Creatine is a compound synthesized in your liver and kidneys to serve as a source of energy for muscle and brain tissue. While creatine is mainly stored in your muscles, as it is metabolized, a small portion of it is converted into *creatinine.* In turn, this breakdown product is transported to your kidneys, filtered from your blood, and removed from your body through your urine. For this reason, a blood creatinine test is a good measure of kidney function, particularly when considered alongside the results of a BUN test. Since creatine and creatinine are associated with muscle, and as men tend to have more muscle than women, men also tend to have higher creatinine levels. Creatine dietary supplements are sometimes used in sports nutrition. If you take creatine supplements, be sure to let your doctor know before you have your blood tested.

BUN/Creatinine Ratio

The results of the blood urea nitrogen and creatinine blood tests are used to calculate the ratio of BUN to creatinine. This is an important ratio to know, as it provides a more accurate picture of kidney health than either test might on its own. This ratio, however, is not typically included in your test results unless your blood urea nitrogen reading or creatinine level is abnormal. If your ratio is high or low, it may indicate kidney dysfunction or other medical conditions. In this case, your doctor will order more comprehensive testing to determine the source of the problem.

Glomerular Filtration Rate (GFW)

While BUN and creatinine levels are crucial in the assessment of kidney health, they may ultimately be insufficient if kidney disease is suspected or has already developed. This fact is why calculating your *glomerular filtration rate* (GFR) is so important. This calculation reflects the amount of blood in your kidneys that is filtered each minute and generally correlates with your urinary output. A glomerular filtration rate below a certain level indicates kidney dysfunction. Your GFR will be calculated by your doctor in cases of *chronic kidney disease* (CKD), diabetes, heart disease, high blood pressure, or family history of chronic kidney disease. Your doctor may also wish to calculate your glomerular filtration rate in cases of frequent urinary tract infections or urinary blockages.

■ THE HEPATIC FUNCTION PANEL YOUR LIVER HEALTH

The *hepatic function panel* determines how well your liver is functioning by measuring levels of different proteins produced or processed by your liver, including albumin and globulin, as well as liver enzymes.

Total Protein

The *total protein* count of the hepatic panel is determined by adding up the amount of albumin and globulin proteins in your blood. Total protein is an important measurement, as it is a determining factor of your nutritional status and aids in the diagnosis of both kidney disease and liver disease. It is also used to gauge the strength of your immune system and investigate the cause of *edema*, which refers to fluid buildup that leads to swelling of ankles and other areas of your body.

Albumin

Made by your liver, *albumin* is the protein responsible for keeping the fluid portion of your blood contained within your blood vessels. Another one of its important roles is to bind to bilirubin, free fatty acids, hormones such as thyroxin and cortisol, nutrients such as calcium and magnesium, as well as pharmaceuticals, which allows these substances to travel throughout your body via your bloodstream. Elevated albumin levels are typically related to dehydration, although other possible causes include low stomach acid, digestive tract inflammation, kidney or liver disease, malnutrition, use of certain medications, vitamin A deficiency, and *pregnancy eclampsia,* a rare condition that can cause seizures during pregnancy.

Globulin

Globulin includes carrier proteins, enzymes, clotting factors, and, predominantly, antibodies. The three main groups of globulins include *alpha globulins, beta globulins,* and *gamma globulins.* Alpha and beta globulins are primarily transport proteins. Gamma globulins are mainly comprised of antibodies, or immunoglobulins. White blood cells, specifically B lymphocytes, produce immunoglobulins in response to infection or allergic reaction.

Albumin/Globulin (A/G) Ratio

The ratio of albumin to globulin, or *A/G ratio,* is used to determine whether or not your protein count is outside the normal range. A high A/G ratio may indicate a lack of gamma globulins, suggesting a compromised immune system. It may also be caused by an underactive thyroid gland. Whether your A/G ratio is determined to be high or low, your doctor will want to do a few follow-up tests to determine the cause of this abnormal result.

Bilirubin

Bilirubin is an orange-yellow compound that appears as a normal byproduct of aging red blood cells being broken down by your spleen. Bilirubin is ultimately released into your bile and stored in your gallbladder. Eventually, it is excreted from your body through your stool. When your liver is damaged or diseased, it will not be able to process bilirubin properly, causing this fluid to accumulate in your blood.

Alanine Aminotransferase (ALAT)

Alanine aminotransferase (ALAT) is an enzyme found predominantly in your liver, although it also occurs in your plasma as well as in your muscles, heart, kidneys, and pancreas. ALT is one of the most important tests used to determine liver damage or disease. When your liver is diseased or damaged, ALAT is released into your bloodstream, causing your blood levels of this enzyme to rise.

Alkaline Phosphatase (ALP)

Also an enzyme, *alkaline phosphatase* (ALP) is found mainly in your liver and bones, with a small amount occurring in your kidneys and intestines. Elevated ALP values are used as tumor markers and to diagnose liver disease. They may also be seen in connection with bone injury, pregnancy, and skeletal growth.

Asparate Aminotransferase (ASAT)

As with ALAT and ALP, *aspartate aminotransferase* (ASAT) is an enzyme found largely in your liver, although some may appear in your heart, skeletal muscle tissue, kidneys, brain, or red blood cells. If one of the aforementioned tissues is damaged, ASAT is released into your bloodstream. In combination with your ALAT count, your ASAT reading is most frequently used to identify liver damage or disease.

Gamma-Glutamyl Transferase (GGT)

The enzyme *gamma-glutamyl transferase* (GGT) is found in numerous tissues throughout your body, including your liver, kidneys, pancreas, spleen, and heart. An elevated GGT reading may suggest liver damage, but consideration of your ALP level is required when attempting to determine the cause of this damage. If both your ALP count and your GGT count are high, then your doctor may narrow down the problem to bile duct disease or liver disease. If your ALP count is high but your GGT reading is not, then your doctor may suspect bone disease. GGT is also very sensitive to alcohol use, so an elevated GGT reading may simply be the result of alcohol consumption.

■ THE COMPLETE BLOOD COUNT (CBC) PANEL

Lab values measured in the *complete blood count* (CBC) panel include red blood cells, white blood cells, platelets, and hemoglobin. Levels of these biomarkers give insight into your vitality and energy, immune system health, and cardiovascular health.

Red Blood Cells (RBCs)

As discussed in the previous chapter, your red blood cells transport oxygen throughout your body while also bringing carbon dioxide to your lungs for you to exhale. They account for 40 to 45 percent of your blood's volume. An elevated RBC reading may occur as the result of low oxygen levels, or when your kidneys release too much of the hormone *erythropoietin,* which promotes RBC production in your bone marrow. A decrease in blood plasma may also lead to high levels of RBCs. These processes may be triggered by a number of different conditions, including bone marrow disorders, lung disease, cardiovascular disease, dehydration, kidney cancer, living at high altitudes, and certain medications.

Hemoglobin

This iron-containing protein in red blood cells binds to oxygen, allowing its transport throughout your body. It also helps move carbon dioxide back to your lungs and plays a role in maintain the shape of your red blood cells. While hemoglobin and RBC counts are interconnected, your red blood cells may still contain unequal amounts of hemoglobin—which means that if your RBC count is normal, you may still have a higher- or lower-than-normal concentration of hemoglobin in your blood. Although routine, hemoglobin tests may also be used to determine the severity of anemia and bleeding disorders.

Hematocrit

Hematrocrit refers to the proportion of your total blood volume that consists of red blood cells. It is not the same as your RBC level. Rather, it is expressed as a percentage, and depends on both the number and size of your red blood cells. The proportion of your red blood cells in relation to the proportions of other cells present in your blood, and whether you have too many or too few RBCs, is reflected in your hematocrit value. This value is needed in order to carry out an accurate assessment of anemia and other blood disorders. Your doctor will also reference this test when trying to determine if you are dehydrated or have a chronic disease or underlying malignancy.

Mean Corpuscular Volume (MCV)

Mean corpuscular volume (MCV) refers to the measurement of the average volume, or size, of your red blood cells. A mean corpuscular volume that is above the normal range is known as *macrocytosis,* or high MCV. A mean corpuscular volume that is below the normal range is known *microcytosis,* or low MCV. MCV values are generally used to differentiate and diagnose various types of anemia.

Mean Corpuscular Hemoglobin (MCH)

Your *mean corpuscular hemoglobin* (MCH) value notes the average amount of hemoglobin contained in a red blood cell. *Hyperchromia* refers to an elevated MCH reading, while *hypochromia* refers to a low MCH value. When you have anemia, your MCH level can help your doctor determine the type of anemia from which you are suffering, as well as its level of severity.

Mean Corpuscular Hemoglobin Concentration (MCHC)

Although closely related, your *mean corpuscular hemoglobin concentration* (MCHC) and your MCH are distinct measurements. Your MCH count represents the average amount of hemoglobin in just one of your red blood cells, while your MCHC number reflects the hemoglobin concentration in a given unit of packed red blood cells in your blood. As with your MCV and MCH values, your MCHC count can help your doctor better assess anemia and other blood disorders.

Platelets

Although they represent only about 20 percent of the size of a red blood cell and a small fraction of your blood in total, platelets have a very important function. They help blood clump and clot around the site of a blood vessel injury, plugging the hole, provided it is not too large. An elevated platelet count may be the result of *thrombocythemia,* a condition in which the bone marrow cells responsible for the production of platelets overproduce these cell fragments.

White Blood Cells (WBCs)

As previously discussed, white blood cells (WBCs) make up 2 percent of your blood and are a marker of the health of your immune system. An elevated WBC count usually indicates the presence of infection in the body, but it may also be caused by lifestyle factors such as strenuous exercise or eating too many refined carbohydrates and sugars. It may also be caused by allergies, bone marrow disorders, severe stress, smoking, thyroid conditions, or tissue damage.

■ HORMONES

As they play an integral role in your reproductive wellness and affect numerous other aspects of your health, certain types of hormones in your body should be periodically tested, especially if you are an adult, although they may not always be included in your routine blood test. These hormones include DHEA, estrogen, progesterone, and testosterone. Although it is not a hormone, if you are male, your doctor may wish to include a prostate-specific antigen (PSA) test along with the previous evaluations, as it measures a related protein. In addition, hormones involved in metabolism, including the thyroid hormones and cortisol (the stress hormone), should also be tested.

DHEA

Predominantly produced in your adrenal glands, *dehydroepiandrosterone,* more commonly called DHEA, serves as a precursor to the sex hormones testosterone and estrogen. DHEA is also a building block of the stress hormone cortisol and supports immune system function. It can also increase insulin sensitivity, enhance fat metabolism, and act as an antioxidant. DHEA appears in your blood predominantly in the form of *dehydroepiandrosterone sulfate* (DHEAS), which remains in your bloodstream longer than free DHEA. A routine blood test will generally measure your DHEAS level. Elevated DHEA may be caused by adrenal tumors, *hyperplasia* (adrenal swelling), or *polycystic ovary syndrome*. It may also be caused by the use of DHEA supplements. To avoid any unwarranted concern about elevated levels, be sure to tell your doctor if you are using any such supplement.

Estrogen

Estrogen is a group of steroid hormones known primarily for their role in sexual development and reproduction. Adult women typically have significantly higher amounts of estrogen than men, particularly during reproductive age. The three main forms of estrogen are *estrone* (E1), *estradiol* (E2), and *estriol* (E3). Estriol is normally the weakest estrogen, and is produced in meaningful amounts only in pregnant women. Estradiol, the most potent form, is the main estrogen in women during their reproductive years. It is also present in males as a derivative of testosterone. Finally, estrone increases in females during menopause to become the predominant estrogen in postmenopausal women. As a woman's ovaries lose the ability to make estradiol, her adrenal glands, liver, and fat cells compensate by producing estrone. The problem is that metabolized estrone can be harmful, and elevated levels can increase the risk of estrogen-related cancers such as breast cancer. Because estrone may be secreted by fat cells, higher than normal amounts may be found in overweight individuals. While they remain fairly constant in men, normal ranges for total estrogen levels in women vary considerably depending on stage of life. They also fluctuate during a woman's menstrual cycle.

Progesterone

Progesterone is a hormone known mainly for its role in conception, pregnancy, and the regulation of a woman's menstrual cycle. Produced in the ovaries, adrenal glands, and the placentas of pregnant women, progesterone also supports bone density, protects against the proliferation of breast and uterine cells, and acts as a coating for the nerve fibers of the brain, reducing *hyperexcitability,* which refers to spontaneous muscular activity. A female's progesterone levels rise and fall according to the stages of her life. While men also synthesize a small amount of this hormone, it is much less important than testosterone when it comes to sexual maturity. Synthetic forms of progesterone, known as *progestins,* are widely used in birth control pills and hormone replacement therapy. Natural progesterone levels are suppressed in women who take synthetic forms, so blood tests are inaccurate in these cases. Otherwise, a blood test is usually administered twenty-one days after the start of a woman's period, if she is still menstruating.

Testosterone

Testosterone is ten times more abundant in men. It is primarily associated with male sexual development, but it also plays a role in the brain function, muscle mass, fat distribution, and energy levels of both sexes. Testosterone is typically attached to a protein in the bloodstream and known as *bound testosterone.* When this hormone is unattached, it is known as *free testosterone,* which is the form most available for use by the body. Generally, a blood test will measure the combination of both types of testosterone, called *total testosterone.* Low testosterone levels may lead to a number of symptoms, including erectile dysfunction, changes in mood, fatigue, sleep disturbances, high blood pressure, low libido, muscle atrophy, joint aches and pains, increased body fat (particularly belly fat), loss of body hair, poor concentration, and blood sugar imbalance.

Prostate-Specific Antigen (PSA)

Located below the bladder in men, the *prostate* is a small gland that produces and releases the liquid component of semen and helps discharge sperm during ejaculation. *Prostate-specific antigen* (PSA) is one of the proteins synthesized by prostate cells. Although it is not a hormone, it may be used as a screening marker for prostate cancer, although this practice has become controversial because it can lead to unnecessary follow-up procedures. Still, many doctors rely on this test as a screening for at-risk males.

Ordinarily, there is a small amount of PSA in a man's blood. Aging, however, can bring about prostate problems, such as enlarged prostate or even prostate cancer. These conditions cause PSA levels to rise as this protein attempts to suppress the growth of prostate cells. Clinicians look at the rate of change in PSA between two readings for evidence of early signs of prostate problems. If your PSA reading suddenly jumps within six months to a year, your doctor may require further testing or examination.

Thyroid Hormones

The *thyroid gland* produces hormones that influence metabolism, energy production, weight control, nerve and gastrointestinal health, nutrient absorption, and oxygen use. Initiated by *thyroid-stimulating hormone* (TSH) from the pituitary gland, thyroid hormone production includes the active hormone *triiodothyronine* (T_3) and the inactive hormone *thyroxine* (T_4), which may be converted into T_3. In addition to a TSH count, thyroid hormone measurements may include levels of total T_3 and T_4, as well as free T_3 and T_4. Free levels refer to the amount of circulating hormone available for use by your cells, while total levels also include the amount of hormone bound to proteins. Typically, free T_3 and T_4 readings are considered more reliable indicators of thyroid disturbances than total readings. Elevated thyroid hormone levels are known as *hyperthyroidism*, while low levels are known as *hypothyroidism*.

Cortisol

Cortisol is a steroid hormone made in your adrenal glands. It increases blood sugar, suppresses your immune system, fights inflammation, decreases bone formation, and helps metabolize fat, protein, and carbohydrates when released in appropriate amounts. It is frequently referred to as the "stress hormone," as it is released in response to both physical and psychological stress. Chronic stress, however, can lead to the creation of too much cortisol in your system, which may result in a variety of problems in your body. Elevated cortisol levels can block the growth of nerve cells in your brain and damage your brain's memory center, known as the *hippocampus,* which may even shrink when high cortisol and low DHEA levels occur together. High cortisol levels may also be caused by adrenal disorders, eating disorders, oral contraceptives, physical activity, pituitary tumors, or pregnancy.

■ IMPORTANT OPTIONAL TESTS

Although not typically measured unless requested by the patient, or if a standard blood test shows an abnormality that requires a more in-depth analysis, blood counts of four additional substances can provide a more complete picture of heart health, immunity, calcium absorption, blood sugar regulation, and a number of other vital processes. These measurements include homocysteine, C-reactive protein (CRP), vitamin D, and magnesium levels.

Homocysteine

Homocysteine is a byproduct of normal protein metabolism, formed from the conversion of the amino acid *methionine.* Since high levels of homocysteine is not a good thing for your health, your body has a built-in mechanism to convert it partially back into methionine and other beneficial, nontoxic amino acids. If, however, this process is somehow disrupted, homocysteine will accumulate in your bodily fluids and tissues and have serious ramifications to your health. The most well-known of these consequences includes an increased risk of cardiovascular disease.[6,7] In fact, homocysteine can be part of your comprehensive lipid profile, which is used to evaluate your total cardiovascular risk. This lab value may also be measured to determine whether your body has a sufficient amount of B vitamins. High homocysteine levels can also lead to depression, fibromyalgia, Alzheimer's disease, or vascular dementia.[8,9,10]

C-Reactive Protein (CRP)

C-reactive protein (CRP) is another lab included in your complete heart risk assessment, as a high reading is usually a sign of inflammation, which research has shown to be correlated with conditions such as heart disease, stroke, and peripheral artery disease.

Vitamin D

Vitamin D has received a lot of attention in recent years due to the growing amount of research on its health benefits. Vitamin D is crucial to heart health, immunity, calcium absorption, and insulin regulation, and may lower the risk of certain medical conditions, including hypertension, osteoporosis, some autoimmune disorders, and even certain types of cancer. Although more and more doctors recommend this test to their patients, vitamin D is still usually measured only when calcium readings are high, or when a person has a condition that may lead to low vitamin D levels.

Magnesium

Magnesium is an essential nutrient that, similarly to vitamin D, takes part in a wide range of functions in the body. Unfortunately, most Americans do not take in sufficient amounts of this mineral, as the standard diet in the United States is instead overloaded with refined sugars and saturated fats—substances that actually increase the body's magnesium requirement. Keeping an eye on magnesium levels through regular blood tests, therefore, can help you maintain proper metabolism, bone formation, and blood sugar regulation, in addition to other basic physiological processes.

CONCLUSION

Although you still need your doctor to interpret the results of your blood tests accurately, hopefully this chapter has provided you with valuable insight into the various components that make up the typical panels of a blood test, as well as useful information on a few blood readings that aren't as commonly taken but may help provide a clearer view of your health status. Remember, in addition to listening to your body's cues, blood tests are one of the best ways to learn whether your diet, lifestyle, and medication (if applicable) are serving you well.

3

How Your Body Cleanses Your Blood

As discussed in Chapter 1, humans are exposed to a great many harmful substances as a result of modern living. These substances include heavy metals, pesticides, industrial compounds and byproducts, medications, and cosmetic additives. Toxins that are foreign to the human biological system are known as *external*, or *exogenous*, toxins. Substances that are naturally produced within the human body that can accumulate to dangerous levels are called *internal*, or *endogenous*, toxins. This chapter will discuss both types of toxins and explain the processes through which your body attempts to rid itself of them.

EXTERNAL TOXINS

For the purposes of this book, external toxins will be split into two groups: heavy metals and other chemical toxins. The following section will describe these substances, list their most common sources in your everyday environment, and detail the ways in which your body detoxifies itself in response to exposure to them.

Heavy Metals

Heavy metals are mineral elements with relatively high atomic weights. Although this fact will not be very meaningful to anyone other than chemists, a more relevant fact is that heavy metals do not tend to contribute nutritional value—as would be the case with other minerals such as calcium and zinc. Rather, heavy metals can have a very negative impact on your health and well-being if they build up in your body.

Heavy metals are fairly widespread, being found in the soil where food grows, in air pollution, and as a byproduct of manufacturing industries. Although your body is capable of processing and eliminating small amounts of heavy metals, as is the case with most toxins, excessive accumulation of these substances can make it difficult for your body to handle them in a timely manner. Of the heavy metals commonly found in our modern environment, those that disrupt the human system most include lead, mercury, cadmium, arsenic, nickel, and aluminum. These heavy metals may accumulate in organs such as the brain and kidneys, as well as in the immune system, where they can severely disrupt normal function.[1,2,3,4,5]

In addition to being found in industrial settings, heavy metals often crop up in places much closer to home—the solder on copper pipes, pesticide sprays, and cooking utensils, all of which may contain lead; cigarette smoke, which may be laced with cadmium and lead; contaminated fish, latex paints, and cosmetics, which have been known to have concerning mercury contents; and even antacids and possibly some forms of cookware, which often consist of a certain amount of aluminum.[6]

Potential early symptoms of heavy metal toxicity include headache, fatigue, muscle pain, indigestion, tremors, constipation, anemia, pallor, dizziness, and poor coordination. Even if you are suffering from a mild case of heavy metal buildup in your body, you will display an impaired ability to think or concentrate. The severity of these symptoms typically increases as your body's burden of heavy metals increases.[7]

Other Chemical Toxins

Simply put, other chemical toxins consist of all external toxins that are not heavy metals. Their sources include chemicals that are used in, or created as a byproduct of, manufacturing, agriculture, and other types of industry. You may ingest these chemicals through food or beverages (or through some of the highly refined products that pass for food or beverages), absorb them through topically applied cosmetics or body care products, inhale them by choice (e.g., tobacco) or through airborne pollutants, and swallow or inject them in the form of certain pharmaceuticals (legal or otherwise).

There are simply too many chemical toxins in the environment to discuss them all adequately in this section. Focus will be placed on the various types that are generally dealt with by the liver and make up the following subcategories: solvents (e.g., cleaning materials, formaldehyde, toluene, and benzene), drugs, alcohol, pesticides (e.g., chlordane, organophosphates), herbicides, food additives (e.g., artificial colors, flavors, and preservatives), as well as PCBs (polychlorinated biphenyls) and phthalates (from plastics). Exposure to certain chemicals in these substances can cause a broad range of symptoms. Among the most common psychological and neurological symptoms are depression, headaches, mental confusion, mental illness (such as dementia), paresthesia, abnormal nerve reflexes, as well as other symptoms associated with an impaired nervous system function, such as muscle weakness. Respiratory tract allergies and increased rates for many cancers may also occur.[8,9,10,11,12,13,14]

INTERNAL TOXINS

As a natural consequence of normal metabolism, your body generates substances, including certain microbial compounds and breakdown products of protein metabolism, which may become harmful to your health if allowed to accumulate in your system. At the risk of sounding like a broken record, your body is made to process these internal toxins, but when there is an overabundance of them, taking care of these substances becomes difficult, and problems may arise.

Microbial Compounds

I am sure you are familiar with the probiotic bacteria that reside in your gut. In short, these are the "friendly" bacteria that you typically find in yogurt and certain supplements. They serve important roles in health, which include helping to metabolism certain food items, promoting immune responses, and even involvement in the production of certain neurotransmitters such as serotonin, which benefits mental health. Likewise, certain yeasts also reside in your gut, including *Candida albicans*. While their role in human health is not entirely clear, there does seem to be a particular balance between them and probiotic bacteria.

These microbial organisms have a symbiotic relationship with you, helping your system in certain important functions in exchange for an environment in which to live (your intestines) and nutrients to flourish. Like any other organism, however, they also have metabolic processes that result in waste products and cellular debris. Examples of these microbial waste compounds include endotoxins (toxins that reside inside certain bacterial cells and are released when these cells are disrupted), exotoxins (toxins secreted by bacterial cells), toxic amines (toxic derivatives of ammonia), toxic derivatives of bile, and various carcinogenic, or cancer-causing, substances. Unfortunately, these compounds may be absorbed into your bloodstream, resulting in significant disturbances in your bodily functions.

Microbial compounds generated in the gut have been implicated in a wide variety of illnesses, including liver disease, Crohn's disease, ulcerative colitis, thyroid disease, psoriasis, lupus erythematosus, pancreatitis, allergies, asthma, and a number of immune disorders. In fact, antibodies form against these microbial compounds and can incorrectly react with your body's own tissues. This reaction, in turn, can contribute to the development of autoimmune diseases such as rheumatoid arthritis, myasthenia gravis, diabetes, pernicious anemia, and autoimmune thyroiditis. Your immune system and liver are responsible for dealing with the toxic substances that are absorbed from the gut.[15]

Breakdown Products of Protein Metabolism

Proteins from your diet, as well as various proteins within your body, are ultimately broken down and metabolized. This occurs as part of digestion (thanks to the hydrochloric acid in your stomach and enzymes in your intestines), which breaks down complex proteins into their component amino acids, and cellular metabolism, which processes amino acids, yielding end products, or breakdown products, of protein metabolism, including ammonia and urea. When your body is already dealing with an overabundance of toxins from other sources, or when it simply isn't functioning up to par due to poor diet, illness, or other lifestyle factors, these breakdown products are not processed and eliminated as efficiently as they should be. (In most cases, ammonia and other breakdown products of protein metabolism are eliminated by your kidneys.) In turn, they may accumulate in your body, which may cause significant health problems. For example, elevated ammonia levels may result in muscle weakness, fatigue, or other symptoms of liver or kidney damage. If left untreated, elevated blood ammonia can affect brain tissue, leading to symptoms such as confusion and delirium (rapid change in cognitive function).

HOW YOUR BODY ELMINATES INTERNAL AND EXTERNAL TOXINS

While it may be incredibly disheartening to hear about the numerous and seemingly unavoidable sources of exposure to toxins and the ways in which these substances can negatively affect your body, or that your body naturally generates byproducts and waste that could harm you, there is some good news. Fortunately, your body has certain mechanisms of detoxification that allow it to rid itself of both exogenous and endogenous toxins. Essentially, it eliminates these troublesome materials either by neutralizing them or by directing them into your urine or feces to be excreted from your body. (To a lesser degree, these substances may also be excreted through your mucous membranes, lungs, and skin).

When your body is unable to eliminate toxins effectively and they begin to build up in your system, they are often stored in fat or bone. Your major organs of detoxification are your liver, intestines, kidneys, and skin. The roles of your skin and kidneys are relatively simple in comparison to the cleansing mechanisms associated with your liver and intestines. Your skin excretes certain toxins such as DDT and, to a limited extent, heavy metals such as lead and mercury through your sweat. Your kidneys utilize your urine to rid your body of many other toxins, although most fat-soluble toxins must first be made water-soluble by your liver before being excreted through your urine. Fat-soluble toxins, as the term suggests, are toxins that can dissolve in fat. They are absorbed along with fat and are stored in your body's fatty tissue. Water-soluble toxins, as their name suggests, are toxins that can dissolve in water. Due to the fact that they can dissolve in water, they do not get trapped in your fat cells and are easily eliminated from your body.

As described in the following section, the complex work of detoxification is done primarily by the liver and secondarily through the intestines.[16] The remainder of this chapter is dedicated to explaining this process.

Detoxification by Your Liver

Water-soluble toxins, such as lead, can pass through your body unchanged and be eliminated in your stool, sweat, or urine. Fat-soluble toxins, such as trichloroethane (a form of chloroform used as an industrial solvent), however, cannot be excreted without undergoing metabolic transformation (detoxification) in your liver so that they may become water-soluble. Liver cells have sophisticated mechanisms to break down potentially toxic substances, including both internal and external compounds. Every drug, chemical, pesticide, and hormone is broken down via two detoxification stages in your liver, which are known as *phase I* and *phase II*.[17,18,19]

Phase I

As you can see, while water-soluble toxins are fairly easy for your body to rid itself of, fat-soluble toxins required more work. This is because fat-soluble toxins first need to be converted into a water-soluble form before your body can dispose of them. This conversion starts in your liver with phase I of the detoxification process, which involves the use of certain enzymes known as cytochrome P450 enzymes. These liver enzymes are involved in changing the structure of the fat-soluble toxin in such a way that another substance can attach itself to it (phase II), allowing this toxin to become water-soluble. Some toxins already have the right structure, so they can bypass phase I and go right to phase II—although this is not the case for the majority of harmful compounds. Unfortunately, phase I generates free radicals, which means there is greater potential for cellular damage during this stage.[20,21]

Phase II

Phase II involves the attachment, or coupling, of a water-soluble substance, which has been internally produced by or taken into your body from your external environment, to a toxin, creating what is known as a *conjugated* substance. This attachment makes the toxic molecule more water-soluble, less harmful, and easier to get rid of.

During phase II, fat-soluble toxins, now structurally changed thanks to phase I, are attached to molecules such as glucuronic acid, sulfate, and glutathione, which your body may make or which may come from food sources. Now these toxins are ready to be excreted. If the molecules are large, they may be excreted through your bile. As described in Chapter 1, these conjugated toxins hitch a ride on your bile, which is secreted by your liver to aid in fat digestion, and then move from your liver to your gallbladder to your intestines, at which point they may be excreted in your fecal matter. If the molecules are smaller, they may be excreted in your urine.[22,23]

Dependent upon its type, each toxin is processed along one of six possible pathways during phase II. Each pathway relates to the substance to which the toxin is attached after passing through phase I. The six phase II pathways are as follows:[24,25,26,27,28]

1. Acetylation. Conjugation of toxins with acetyl-CoA (a derivative of pantothenic acid, also known as vitamin B_5) is the primary method by which your body eliminates a type of antibacterial agent known as sulfa drugs. This system appears to be especially sensitive to genetic variation, with those having a poor acetylation mechanism being far more susceptible to sulfa drugs and other antibiotics.

2. Amino Acid Conjugation. Several amino acids, including glycine, taurine, and glutamine, are used in this detoxification pathway, combining with and neutralizing substances such as benzoic acid (a preservative). Glycine is the most commonly utilized substance in phase II amino acid conjugation. Unfortunately, amino acid conjugation does not tend to work as effectively in patients suffering from hepatitis, liver disorders, carcinomas, chronic arthritis, hypothyroidism, toxemia of pregnancy, or excessive chemical exposure, who all tend to have poorly functioning amino acid conjugation systems. For example, in people with liver disease, benzoic acid is detoxified at only half the rate that it is in healthy adults.

3. Glucuronidation. Glucuronidation occurs when glucuronic acid, a natural acid found in foods such as apples and grapefruit, combines with a toxin. Many commonly prescribed drugs, including morphine, lorazepam (Ativan), and codeine, are detoxified through this pathway. It also plays a role in the detoxification of aspirin, menthol, vanillin (synthetic vanilla), food additives such as benzoates, and some hormones.

4. Glutathione Conjugation. Glutathione (a tripeptide composed of cysteine, glutamic acid, and glycine) conjugation produces water-soluble compounds, which are then excreted in your urine. The elimination of heavy metals such as mercury and lead is dependent upon your body maintaining adequate levels of glutathione.

5. Methylation. Methylation involves coupling methyl groups with toxins. Methyl groups are compounds naturally found in vitamin B_{12} and folate (vitamin B_9), as well as foods that contain them, such as fish, meat, milk, and eggs—which contain vitamin B_{12}—and leafy green vegetables, citrus fruit, and strawberries— which contain folate. Methylation helps in the detoxification of heavy metals such as mercury and arsenic, and even of certain hormones, including epinephrine (adrenaline).

6. Sulfation. Sulfation is the coupling of toxins with sulfur-containing compounds, which may be found in such foods as garlic, onions, and broccoli, as well as methylsulfonylmethane (MSM) supplements. This pathway is important in the detoxification of several types of drugs, food additives, and, especially, toxins from intestinal bacteria. In addition to helping eliminate these harmful substances from your body, the sulfation pathway is also involved in the regulation of certain hormones, such as thyroid hormones and steroids. Finally, the sulfation pathway is the primary route for the elimination of neurotransmitters, also known as chemical messengers, such as serotonin, which transmits important signals in your nervous system that are connected with mood and appetite control. As a result, any dysfunction in sulfation may contribute to the development of nervous system disorders, including seizures.

Detoxification by Your Intestines

Although your small intestine mainly functions as the site where most nutrients are absorbed by your body, it is also the first site of toxin exposure, and is presented with the largest load of toxins confronting your body. Consequently, it should come as no surprise that there is an additional phase—phase III—of the detoxification process that is highly concentrated in the small intestine. Phase III is known as antiporter activity.[29]

The word "antiporter" seems to suggest activity against the transportation of toxins, but this is not the case at all. It actually means that it redirects transportation of toxins to a different area. For example, rather than allow toxins to be absorbed through the lining of your intestines into your bloodstream, antiporter activity redirects them away from your intestinal lining and back into the "tube" part of your intestines, where they may be ultimately excreted.[30] This antiporter activity is a function of certain proteins, the best known of which is P-glycoprotein.

P-glycoprotein is extensively distributed and expressed throughout your intestinal lining. It is also found in your liver cells, where it pumps toxins into your bile duct, which, in turn, dumps them into your intestines to be excreted by your body. Likewise, P-glycoprotein is found in the cells of your kidney tubules. It pumps toxins into your kidney's urine-carrying ducts for elimination through your urine. P-glycoprotein is also found in the capillary cells that make up your protective blood–brain barrier, which keeps toxins away from your brain, and your blood-testis barrier, which keeps toxins away from your testes.[31] As the antiporter system is responsible for the transport of fat-soluble toxins out of the liver after phase II conjugation, it is referred to as phase III of detoxification.

PHASE III DYSFUNCTION

Phase III dysfunction may occur when inflammation is present, especially if the inflammation is in your gut. Sources of inflammation include inflammatory bowel disease and even something as basic as excessive intake of refined carbohydrates or vegetable oils, which has been associated with elevated levels of inflammation. When phase III is blocked, phase II enzymes do not function as well, and this can ultimately lead to a buildup of toxins in your body. In addition, this accumulation of toxins can cause oxidative damage, which may further impair your body's ability to detoxify itself.[32]

Detoxification Guide

The following guide (Table 3.1) provides an overview of the various organs at play in detoxification, the methods of detoxification with which these organs are associated, and examples of the toxins that are eliminated from your body through these organs.[33]

TABLE 3.1. DETOXIFICATION GUIDE		
Organ	**Detoxification Method**	**Examples of Eliminated Toxins**
Skin	Excretion through sweat	• DDT
		• Heavy metals
Liver	Filtering of the blood	• Bacteria
		• Bacterial products
	Bile secretion	• Cholesterol
		• Hemoglobin breakdown products
	Phase I detoxification	• Many prescription drugs
		• Many over-the-counter drugs
		• Caffeine
		• Hormones
		• Carcinogens from charcoal-broiled meat
		• Some dyes
		• Carbon tetrachloride
		• Insecticides
	Phase II detoxification *Glutathione conjugation*	• Acetaminophen
		• Nicotine
		• Insecticides
	Phase II detoxification *Amino acid conjugation*	• Benzoates (food preservatives)
		• Aspirin

Organ	Detoxification Method	Examples of Eliminated Toxins
Liver (cont.)	Phase II detoxification *Methylation*	• Dopamine (neurotransmitter)
		• Epinephrine (hormone)
	Phase II detoxification *Sulfation*	• Estrogen
		• Some dyes
		• Coumarin
		• Acetaminophen
	Phase II detoxification *Acetylation*	• Sulfonamides (antibiotics)
	Phase II detoxification *Glucuronidation*	• Acetaminophen
		• Morphine
		• Diazepam (sedative)
Intestines	Mucosal detoxification	• Toxins from bowel bacteria
	Excretion through feces	• Toxins excreted in the bile, including most phase II toxins after they have been processed by your liver (e.g., benzoates, coumarin)
Kidneys	Excretion through urine	• Acetaminophen
		• Nicotine

This table clearly illustrates the previously stated point that your skin and kidneys play relatively simple roles in detoxification next to the work done by your liver and, to a lesser degree, your intestines.

CONCLUSION

There are many exogenous and endogenous toxins, or external and internal toxins, to which your body is exposed on a regular basis. They include heavy metals and other chemical toxins, as well as microbial compounds and breakdown products of protein metabolism. Exposure to these substances can lead to various negative health consequences. (See Chapter 5.) Luckily, your body possesses an extensive detoxification system to process and eliminate these toxins. The operation of this mechanism consists of three phases (phase I, phase II, and phase III), which take place in your liver and intestines, as well as in your kidneys and, to a lesser extent, in your skin. Of course, the total toxic load to which you are exposed, and which your body must work hard to neutralize or excrete, is heavily impacted by what you eat. Certain foods can positively impact your system of blood detoxification, while others can negatively affect this mechanism. The following chapter will discuss this aspect of blood health in greater detail.

PART TWO

What Your Blood Needs

Part Two of this book is all about the vital compounds your blood needs to work properly and keep your body in good health. Chapter 4 focuses on the six major types of nutrients required by your body for energy production, cell growth, and organ function. Chapter 5 provides guidance on choosing the right foods to produce the greatest positive impact on your blood, and thus on your well-being. Chapter 6 then discusses the importance of maintaining optimum blood oxygen levels, explains how your blood goes about transporting oxygen throughout your body, and suggests how you can ensure your blood gets plenty of oxygen every day.

4

Understanding Nutrients

Anutrient is a substance that an organism utilizes to maintain its life and grow. This chapter will focus on the six major types of nutrients that your body requires for proper health: carbohydrates, fat, protein, vitamins, minerals, and water. Each of these major nutrients has its own specific function, and they all work together in the production of energy, the promotion of cell growth, and the achievement of proper organ function once absorbed into your bloodstream from the varied forms of nourishment found in food.

The path that these life-sustaining substances take in your body begins in your gastrointestinal tract. Your stomach breaks down the foods you eat, making their nutrients easier for your intestines to absorb, and moves them to your small intestine. Here, the nutrients made available from your food use tiny finger-like projections known as *villi,* which are found along your small intestine's inner wall, to enter your bloodstream. (Most nutrients are absorbed in your small intestine, but your large intestine also takes in some nutrients. It contains bacteria that help digest any remaining digestible food before your body excretes the waste products of the entire process.)

Your blood carries these nutrients from your intestines to your liver, which breaks them down for easier use by the other tissues of your body. Any harmful byproducts of this mechanism are taken up by your bile, which is produced by your liver, or released into your bloodstream. Those byproducts that are swept up by your bile enter your intestine and exit your body through your stool. Those byproducts that are released into your blood are filtered out by your kidneys and eliminated in your urine. Your liver, in fact, is involved in hundreds of crucial bodily processes, including the production of cholesterol, the storage of excess glucose as glycogen, the regulation of amino acid levels in your blood, the conversion of ammonia into urea (a byproduct of protein metabolism that exits your body through urination), the regulation of blood clotting, and the removal of bacteria from your bloodstream.

As the title of Part 2 of this book suggests, the next few chapters are about the needs of your blood. As nutrients play vital roles in the health of your blood and body, they are a great place to start. To help you better understand nutrients and their importance to your well-being, these substances have been divided into two categories: macronutrients and micronutrients.

MACRONUTRIENTS

As their name suggests, *macronutrients* are required by your body in greater amounts than are micronutrients. They include carbohydrates, fat, protein, and water. Apart from water, these nutrients are broken down by your digestive system so that they may supply energy to your body. This vital transfer of energy is reliant upon a molecule called adenosine triphosphate, or ATP, which is considered the most important molecule in the human body and commonly referred to as the "currency of life," as it stores the fuel you need to function.

To explain, the metabolic process releases energy from macronutrients and generates ATP molecules, which trap this free energy. ATP provides this fuel to cells whenever they require it. When you eat carbohydrates, protein, or fat, these substances are digested and, as a result, converted into bioavailable components—carbohydrates are broken down into sugars, fat is broken down into fatty acids or glycerol, and protein is broken down into amino acids—all of which lead to the release of chemical energy. ATP then helps transfer the energy produced by these reactions to your cells. Your body simply could not function without macronutrients and ATP to supply it with energy.

■ CARBOHYDRATES

Carbohydrates are the most rapidly utilized source of fuel for your body. Once carbohydrates have been digested, the resultant simple sugars, also known as monosaccharides, are absorbed into your bloodstream. These sugars include glucose, fructose, and galactose. Glucose is used right away as your body's most efficient source of energy. Galactose and fructose are metabolised further in your liver to generate glucose and small amounts of other metabolites. They are taken up quickly by your liver to produce glucose, so only small amounts of these sugars are found in your bloodstream at any time. It is thought that the glucose created from fructose and galactose is primarily converted into *glycogen,* the form of glucose that serves as stored energy in your body, instead of released into your blood. In contrast, the glucose immediately received by your body after the breakdown of carbohydrates is transported through your bloodstream to your tissues. At this point, the hormone insulin allows glucose to be taken up by your cells and used as energy.

Because glucose is so important to your body—and, in particular, to your most energy-demanding organ, your brain—your system tries to maintain a steady amount of blood glucose circulating at all times. Any surplus glucose is stored as glycogen in your liver or muscles. The glycogen reserve in your liver is then used to keep your blood sugar from fluctuating too much between meals, while the glycogen reserve in your muscles is typically used during movement. If these reserves are full, however, any excess glucose in your body is turned into fat, which may be considered long-term storage of energy.

Type 2 Diabetes

It goes without saying that the more carbohydrates you eat at one sitting, the more glucose will be released into your blood. Elevated glucose levels in your blood will signal your pancreas to release the hormone insulin. Insulin allows glucose to enter your cells. Without it, glucose will not be able to be turned into energy. When your blood sugar levels are frequently high, your cells may begin to lose their ability to respond to insulin. This is what is known as *type 2 diabetes.* As your body tightly regulates

LOW-CARB/HIGH-PROTEIN DIETING

In an effort to lose weight or lower blood sugar levels (or both), people have been turning to low-carb dieting, which often involves consuming large amounts of animal-derived foods. Once on this diet, most people feel they can eat as much protein-rich animal products as they like, as these foods don't spike blood glucose levels and do not cause them to gain weight as easily as do carbs. There are reasons, however, to take caution with this approach to nutrition.

It is true that when you eat very few carbohydrates and lots of protein, you tend to lose weight. This type of diet actually changes your metabolism from a carb-burning mechanism to a fat-burning one. When your body breaks down fat, molecules known as ketone bodies, or ketones, are one of the byproducts of this metabolic process. These ketones are released into your bloodstream and may be used as an energy source. When your body relies on ketones for energy in the absence of glucose from carbohydrates, it has entered what is known as a state of ketosis. This state helps to suppress your appetite and increases your loss of fluids through urine. (Coincidentally, ketosis can occur in diabetics, who cannot metabolize glucose properly.)

This metabolic state, however, may result in negative consequences to your health in the long-term, despite the fact that it has desirable short-term benefits. One issue in particular is ammonia, a compound that arises from the breakdown of protein in your

your blood sugar, any problems that might affect this regulation, such as diabetes, will likely lead to noticeable changes in your energy levels.

Dietary Fiber

Dietary fiber is an exception when it comes to carbohydrate metabolism, in that your body cannot digest or absorb dietary fiber as it does other carbohydrates. Fiber simply moves through your digestive system and is excreted relatively unchanged in your

intestines. While your liver converts ammonia into *urea*, a compound that may be excreted in your urine, consistently elevated levels of ammonia may overburden this process, leading to a buildup of ammonia in your blood, which can affect your brain tissue and lead to confusion, delirium, and other neurological disorders.

In addition, there is evidence to suggest that the acidic state caused by a high-protein diet may force your body to release calcium from its stores as a buffer, leading to calcium loss in your urine. Calcium loss, understandably, is closely connected to osteoporosis and lack of bone strength.

If your body cannot adequately neutralize this acidic state, it will enter a dangerously acidic state known as ketoacidosis. Ketoacidosis can lead to a coma or even death, but is more commonly associated with diabetics who do not manage their disease than with low-carb/high-protein dieters. The most obvious sign of ketoacidosis is smelly urine or breath that smells like nail polish remover (acetone).

Finally, when you opt for protein-rich animal foods, you are often not getting enough fruit and vegetables in your diet. Fruit and vegetables are the wonderful dietary sources of antioxidants, certain vitamins and minerals, and fiber, all of which help prevent disease. Animal-derived foods, on the other hand, are typically high in saturated fat, which has been linked to heart disease, diabetes, and several types of cancer. Meat also lacks fiber, which is crucial to your well-being.

stool. As such, fiber does not act as a source of energy for your major bodily functions, although it is now understood that dietary fiber does, in fact, supply energy to the "friendly" bacteria in your large intestine, also known as *probiotics.* Through a process known as *fermentation,* these bacteria actually feed on a portion of the dietary fiber as it passes through your colon. Research suggests that colonies of healthy gut bacteria may benefit your immune system and even protect against certain cancers, heart disease, and arthritis. Fermentation also produces gases, which is the reason that a high-fiber diet can lead to flatulence and bloating.

There are two varieties of fiber: soluble and insoluble. *Soluble fiber* dissolves in water to form a gel-like substance that softens your fecal matter and slows its movement through your digestive system. In doing so, it increases your body's opportunity to absorb nutrients from food while also making you feel fuller for a longer period of time, which may help if you are trying to lose weight. It also slows the rate at which your body absorbs glucose, thus lowering blood sugar level. Another of soluble fiber's important biological effects is its role in reducing your blood cholesterol level. When soluble fiber binds to bile acids in your intestines, your liver must produce more bile. In order to do so, it requires cholesterol, which it takes from your blood. Including an adequate amount of this type of fiber in your diet, therefore, can aid in the regulation of your cholesterol levels and lower your risk of heart disease.

Soluble fibers also ferment in your large intestine, creating fatty acids that can help regulate your blood sugar, boost your immune cell production, and lower the level of LDL cholesterol in your blood. Finally, fermentation of soluble fiber promotes a healthy pH balance in your large intestine while also encouraging the production of friendly bacteria in your colon.[1] While both fibers may be found in any fiber-rich food, soluble fiber may be found in substantial amounts in oatmeal, fruit, vegetables, nuts, beans, and flaxseeds.

Insoluble fiber, as its name suggests, cannot be dissolved in water. It acts as a bulking agent for your stool, preventing constipation. Since constipation can lead to a myriad of health difficulties, including hemorrhoids and diverticulitis, and is the most reported gastrointestinal complaint in the United States, it is clear that an adequate intake of insoluble fibers is an important part of maintaining good health.[2]

Diverticulitis, in fact, is one of the most common intestinal disorders in Western society, its risk increasing with age. This condition occurs when small pouches in your digestive tract (typically in your colon), known as *diverticula,* become inflamed or infected, leading to symptoms such as abdominal pain, nausea, and fever. The cause of diverticula remains unknown, although the formation of these tiny sacs has been associated with a low-fiber diet. Even if you already have diverticula, research has shown that insoluble fiber can help control episodes of diverticulitis by encouraging stool to pass easily through your large intestine.

Whole wheat flour, whole grains, wheat bran, oat bran, beans, fruits with edible skins, cabbage, lettuce, bell peppers, and onions are all good sources of insoluble fiber, although the fiber found in wheat and oat bran has been shown to be the most effective food source of this substance.

Whether dietary fiber is promoting a smooth process of stool elimination and sweeping undesirable chemical compounds from your body or fermenting in your colon and producing friendly bacteria in your intestinal tract as a result, this type of carbohydrate is indispensible in terms of your overall well-being. If you feel the need to increase your intake of dietary fiber, recommendations of how to do so include eating fruits whole instead of drinking juices, opting for whole grain products when you are planning your meals, grabbing raw vegetables as a snack instead of junk food, and eliminating meat from your menu at least twice a week by using a substitute such as legumes in your meat-based recipes if possible. When you begin to eat more fiber, however, do so gradually and be sure to increase your water intake as well.

■ FAT

Fats, also known as lipids, are the most concentrated form of energy in the diet. Although fat contains approximately twice the amount of energy per gram as carbohydrates, your body has a much more difficult time using it as fuel, which is why the glucose attained from carbohydrates is your system's go-to energy source. Your metabolic mechanism breaks down fat into fatty acids and glycerol, which are absorbed into your blood. Many of your body's cells may use glucose or fatty acids to produce ATP and receive energy.

Your liver also takes these fatty acids and uses them to generate molecules called *ketone bodies*, or *ketones*. Whereas glucose was once considered your brain's only means of energy, research has shown that when this simple sugar is in short supply—such as when you are fasting, following a low-carb diet, or exercising for a prolonged period of time—your brain may use ketones as fuel instead. In this sense, ketones may be seen as a backup source of energy for your brain. They may also serve as a backup supply of energy for your heart and muscles as well.

There is some debate on the benefits of the human body's use of glucose versus ketones as means of fuel, with some low-carb adherents suggesting that we should rely on ketones over glucose more than we presently do. The repercussions of entering a state in which your body places a greater reliance on ketones for energy, known as *ketosis,* are not fully understood, however. Ketones have demonstrated the ability to suppress appetite, which is very helpful if you are trying to lose weight. But high ketone levels in your blood increase your blood's acidity, which may lead to illness. In particular, those with diabetes should avoid entering ketosis in order to prevent kidney or liver damage.

In terms of the glycerol derived from fat, your body can convert it into glucose, but because glycerol makes up such a small part of fat, it is relatively inconsequential in the grand scheme of energy production. It was once thought that fatty acids could not be converted into glucose, but in recent years scientists have gained a more complex understanding of fatty acid metabolism, and it seems that fatty acids can lead to the synthesis of new glucose. Pathways have been discovered by which a derivative of fatty acids, a ketone known as *acetone,* may be converted into glucose. These pathways are so convoluted and complex, however, that this process does not factor into the overall discussion of energy production either.

In addition to providing energy, fat acts as a carrier for fat-soluble vitamins A, D, E, and K. These vitamins are essential parts of your daily diet. Fat also plays an important role in the conversion of beta carotene, the red-orange pigment found in many fruits and vegetables, into vitamin A, which promotes eye health and good vision. Vitamin D helps you maintain the strength of your bones and teeth by boosting calcium absorption, vitamin E protects your cells by neutralizing harmful free radicals in your blood, and vitamin K makes sure your blood will clot when necessary. In addition, essential fatty acids linoleic acid and linolenic acid, which cannot be created by your body and therefore must be obtained through your diet, help your body fight inflammation, promote blood clotting, and encourage brain development. Good sources of these essential fatty acids include fatty fish, olive oil, and seeds.

Saturated Fat

Saturated fat gets its name from the fact that its carbon chains hold as many hydrogen atoms as they possibly can, making them saturated with hydrogen atoms. This type of fat is solid at room temperature and may be found in red meat, whole dairy products, coconut oil, baked goods, and countless other snacks common in the average Western diet. Saturated fat is considered harmful to your health, as it can increase LDL cholesterol in your blood, which can lead to heart disease by encouraging the formation of blockages in your arteries. In recent years, however, science has taken another look at saturated fat, with numerous studies suggesting insufficient evidence to link saturated fat to heart disease—although they did suggest that replacing saturated fat with polyunsaturated fat might lower heart disease risk. While recent research shows that the consumption of polyunsaturated fat or high-fiber carbohydrates instead of saturated fat may reduce the occurrence of heart disease, it also suggests that replacing saturated fat with highly processed carbohydrates may lead to a rise in heart disease.

Unsaturated Fat

Unsaturated fat gets its name from the fact that its carbon chains hold fewer hydrogen atoms than do those of saturated fat. It has also been called the "good fat." It may be found in vegetables, nuts, seeds, and fish. There are two kinds of unsaturated fat: monounsaturated fat and polyunsaturated fat. Chemically speaking, these fats earn their names from the number of double bonds of carbon atoms they contain. (Monounsaturated fat has one while polyunsaturated fat has more than one.) Monounsaturated fat is liquid at room temperature. Good sources of monounsaturated fat include olives, olive oil, canola oil, most nuts, peanut oil, and avocados.

The health benefits of monounsaturated fat came to the forefront during the 1960s, when research showed that people in Greece and other Mediterranean countries had a lower rate of heart disease than the general population despite the fact that they ate a high-fat diet. It was then pointed out that the type of fat most eaten in this area of the world was not derived from animals but rather plants, specifically olives. These findings encouraged much interest in olive oil and promoted the healthful style of eating now commonly known as the "Mediterranean diet." Monounsaturated fat has been associated with improved cholesterol levels, making it good for your heart, and may aid in the regulation of insulin and blood sugar in your blood.

Polyunsaturated fats are essential to the creation of healthy cell membranes and nerve coverings. They also play a role in blood clotting, muscle movement, and healthy skin. The two major kinds of polyunsaturated fat are omega-3 fatty acids and omega-6 fatty acids.

Omega-3 fatty acids reduce your blood pressure, boost your HDL cholesterol levels, and lower your triglycerides. These actions protect you against having a heart attack or stroke. Due to their anti-inflammatory properties, omega-3s may also help wean rheumatoid arthritis patients off their corticosteroid medications. Good sources of omega-3 fatty acids are fatty fish such as sardines and salmon, walnuts, flaxseeds, and canola oil.

Omega-6 fatty acids have also been linked to healthy heart function and may be found in foods such as safflower oil, corn oil, soybeans and soybean oil, sunflower seeds and sunflower oil, and walnuts. They are also present in fatty fish such as herring, mackerel, tuna, and salmon. Omega-6 fatty acids promote healthy skin, hair growth, bone health, and a healthy metabolism. It must be noted, however, that some omega-6 fatty acids produce inflammation in your body when consumed in high amounts, which is why it is always necessary to balance these fats with enough omega-3 fatty acids, which are anti-inflammatory, in your diet. Unfortunately, the typical American diet, with its high junk food and processed food contents, contains far more omega-6 fatty acids, which may be found in abundance in junk food and processed (which generally contain soybean oil, safflower oil, or corn oil as a main ingredient), than it does omega-3s. It is thought that you should consume omega-6s and omega-3s at a ratio of four to one, respectively, although some recommend a ratio of one to one.

Thankfully, natural, unprocessed foods that contain fat will have all three major types of this macronutrient, and so you should be able to maintain a healthy balance of fats in your blood by simply having a diet predominantly composed of whole foods.

Triglycerides

Triglycerides are stored in the fat cells of your body and actually make up the main component of body fat. Your body generates triglycerides when it is faced with more calories than it requires for immediate use, converting these calories into this fat-related chemical compound. Triglycerides are supposed to provide energy between meals, but they accumulate when unused, which is often the case in the modern world. They have been linked to the thickening of arterial walls, also known as atherosclerosis, and thus are associated with increased risks of heart disease and stroke.

Cholesterol

Cholesterol is a fat-related substance known as a lipoprotein, and while it has gotten a bad rap, it is necessary for good health. It is a normal component of most bodily tissues, especially those of your brain, nervous system, liver, and blood. It is needed to form sex hormones, adrenal hormones, vitamin D, and bile, which is required in the proper digestion of fat. An excessive intake of cholesterol-containing foods, however, can adversely affect your cardiovascular health. The relationship between elevated blood cholesterol levels and heart disease has been well established.[3]

Excessive Fat

As is the case with carbohydrates in your diet, excessive amounts of fat in your diet may lead to abnormal weight gain and obesity if more calories are consumed than required by your body. In addition to obesity, excessive fat consumption will lead to abnormally slow digestion and absorption, resulting in indigestion. Additionally, if a lack of carbohydrates is accompanied by a lack of water in your diet, or if your kidneys are malfunctioning, your system will not be able to metabolize fat completely, leading to serious health complications.[4]

■ PROTEIN

Protein is one of the most important substances when it comes to maintaining good health and vitality. Aside from water, protein is the most plentiful type of molecule in your body. As a major component of all your cells, it may be found throughout your body, including in your organs, hair, and skin, and especially in your muscles. You need protein in your diet to help your body repair itself. It is required to form new blood cells and used to carry signals from one part of your body to another. In addition to being the major source of building materials in your body, protein may be used as a source of heat and energy. Your body will turn to this macronutrient as its main source of energy only when faced with insufficient amounts of carbohydrates and fat to do the job.[5]

Protein is made up of a chain of amino acids, which are also known as the "building blocks of life." When your body digests protein, it is broken down into amino acids, which are then used to form enzymes, which speed up the rate of chemical reactions in your body, aiding in digestion and metabolism; hormones, which are signaling molecules that coordinate countless processes within your body; neurotransmitters, which also act as chemical messengers to relay signals between your nerve cells; and antibodies, which your immune system uses to fight pathogens. Protein molecules also form hemoglobin in your blood, which carries oxygen from your lungs to your other tissues and takes carbon dioxide from your tissues to your lungs.

In addition, protein has a positive impact on weight loss due to its ability to increase levels of the hormone glucagon in your blood, which helps control body fat.[6] Protein effects the release of glucagon. Glucagon inhibits the release of insulin in your system and causes the liver to break down stored glycogen into glucose to use as energy. It also helps liberate free fatty acids from your adipose tissue, or fat, for your body to use as fuel, thus eliminating some of your body fat.

Amino Acids

As amino acids are the building blocks of proteins, protein digestion results in the release of amino acids into your bloodstream.

The human body requires approximately twenty-two amino acids in a specific pattern to make a protein. There are two major kinds of amino acids in your body: essential amino acids, which refer to the amino acids that your body cannot make on its own and therefore must be consumed in your diet; and nonessential amino acids, which your body is able to generate on its own. Finally, there is a category called conditionally essential amino acids, which straddles the proverbial fence between the two main kinds of amino acids.

This type includes the amino acids of which your body cannot always make enough under certain conditions (when you are under stress, for example). The following is a list of these three categories.

Essential Amino Acids

Histidine	Lysine	Threonine
Isoleucine	Methionine	Tryptophan
Leucine	Phenylalanine	Valine

Nonessential Amino Acids

Alanine	Aspartic Acid	Proline
Asparagine	Glutamic Acid	Serine

Conditionally Essential Amino Acids

Arginine	Glutamine
Cysteine	Tyrosine

Once your digestive system has broken down protein into its constituent amino acids, these compounds enter a sort of reserve pool of amino acids circulating in your blood. Your body then takes amino acids from this reserve as needed to create important molecules in your body (enzymes, hormones, neurotransmitters, antibodies, etc.) that transport substances throughout your body and help in growth and repair of your cells. This is why you cannot function properly without an adequate intake of protein in your diet.

When a food contains all essential amino acids in sufficient amounts it is called a "complete protein." Animal-derived foods tend to be complete proteins, while fruits, vegetables, grains, seeds, and legumes tend to lack one or more essential amino acids. You need not be a carnivore, however, to obtain complete proteins in your diet. In fact, the typical American diet, with its over-reliance on animal products, contains far more protein than required— arguably far too much. As long as you eat a healthy combination of plant-based foods, you should get all the complete proteins you need while avoiding the unhealthy aspects of consuming a diet high in animal products.

■ WATER

Water is not only the most abundant macronutrient in your body (accounting for roughly 60-percent of your weight), it is responsible for and involved in nearly every process in your body, including circulation, digestion, absorption, and excretion. Water provides no energy but is the primary transporter of nutrients throughout your system. It participates in chemical reactions; acts as a solvent for vitamins, minerals, amino acids, and glucose; functions as a lubricant and cushion around your joints; acts as a shock absorber in your eyes and spinal cord; and forms the amniotic fluid that nurtures and protects fetuses in the womb. Water helps you maintain a normal body temperature and blood volume and plays an essential role in carrying waste material out of your body.

MICRONUTRIENTS

As previously mentioned, *micronutrients* are known as such because they are required only in small amounts. Nevertheless, they are crucial to your health and well-being. Deficiencies in micronutrients can lead to a number of health problems, including anemia, or weakness (low iron), poor cognitive function (low vitamin B_{12}), muscle spasms and sleep troubles (low magnesium), high blood pressure (low potassium), and osteoporosis (calcium deficiency). Micronutrients are involved in the regulation of your metabolism, heartbeat, cellular pH, and bone density. They foster immune system strength and protect against oxidant-related cellular damage. They help your body produce enzymes, hormones, and other compounds necessary to proper growth and function.

In everyday language, micronutrients are simply known as vitamins and minerals. They include vitamins such as A, the B complex, C, D, E, and K, as well as minerals such as calcium, phosphorus, choline, chromium, copper, iodine, iron, magnesium, manganese, potassium, sodium, chloride, selenium, and zinc.

As long as you eat a balanced diet that includes lots of vegetables, fruit, whole grains, and nuts, you should get a sufficient amount of the micronutrients your body requires to function properly. An easy way to be sure to get the variety of micronutrients you need is to choose colorful fruits and vegetables. Purple grapes, orange carrots, red apples, and leafy greens are all wonderful additions to your daily meal plan. If your plate is colorful, you know you're eating correctly. Try to include at least two or more vegetables at every sitting. Opt for a fruit salad instead of cake or cookies for dessert. Make soups or hearty salads for dinner or lunch. There are so many delicious ways to fill up your plate with micronutrients.

One of the benefits of eating in this way is the fact that your diet will contain plenty of whole foods, which not only supply your body with the micronutrients it requires for good health but also aid in weight loss and the maintenance of a healthy weight. Foods that are high in micronutrients tend to also have high fiber and water contents. As a result, they will make you feel fuller for a longer period of time, making you less likely to indulge in junk food throughout your day.

■ VITAMINS

Being micronutrients, *vitamins* are substances required in minute quantities (micrograms to milligrams) but perform vital functions in your cells and tissues to help you keep your body in good health, promote growth and repair, and prevent various illnesses. Unlike carbohydrates, fat, and protein, vitamins are not a source of energy, although they are associated with the enzymes that release energy from macronutrients.

Vitamins may be divided into two categories: *fat-soluble* and *water-soluble.* These adjectives refer to the way in which vitamins are absorbed by your body and whether they are able to be stored for later use. Fat-soluble vitamins require an accompanying fat source for proper absorption by your body. They can also be stored in your body for extended periods of time. For this reason, the need not be replenished as often as water-soluble vitamins. Fat-soluble vitamins include vitamins A, D, E, and K.

Water-soluble vitamins, on the other hand, do not require fat for absorption. As a result, they are easily lost through urination and the secretion of other bodily fluids. These vitamins include vitamin C and the B complex. They tend to circulate in your blood for only a few hours after being ingested, with the exception of vitamin B_{12}, which may remain in your system for up to a week. Therefore, it is very important to consume sources of water-soluble vitamins every day to stay healthy.

Vitamin A

Vitamin A is important for normal vision, integrity of the epithelial cells (the skin and the cells lining the inner surfaces of the body), gene expression, reproduction, embryonic development, growth, and immune function. Research also suggests that vitamin A may have the ability to stop DNA mutations in cancerous cells.

Vitamin B Complex

While vitamins do not act as a source of fuel for your body, the eight *B vitamins* (B_1, B_2, B_3, B_5, B_6, B_7, B_9, B_{12}—collectively called the "B complex") work together to help your body turn macronutrients into energy, thus indirectly keeping you energized. Specifically, B vitamins are converted into *coenzymes*, which are compounds that are required for enzymes, which promote energy metabolism, to function. In addition, some b vitamins help build new cells to deliver the oxygen and nutrients that permit the energy pathways to function. B–complex vitamins are also intimately involved in the function of the nervous system.

While B vitamins work together, individual B vitamins can benefit your body in particular ways as well. For example, vitamin B_{12} makes hemoglobin, which helps your body fight fatigue by carrying oxygen throughout your blood. Riboflavin, also known as vitamin B_2, has been shown to fight headaches and migraines, muscle cramps, carpal tunnel syndrome, and acne. It may even help prevent cervical cancer.

Vitamin C

One of the chief functions of *vitamin C* in your body is the synthesis of *collagen,* the main protein in connective tissue, which strengthens blood vessel walls, forms scar tissue, and provides the required matrix for bone growth. Vitamin C also acts as an antioxidant, protecting against free radicals and thus cancer, and is also involved in thyroxin (the main hormone in your thyroid gland) synthesis, amino acid metabolism, infection resistance, and iron absorption.

Vitamin D

Vitamin D's primary role in human nutrition is to facilitate the absorption of calcium and phosphorus in the intestinal tract, thereby promoting mineralization of bones. Vitamin D is known as "the sunshine vitamin" due to the fact that ultraviolet rays of the sun convert a cholesterol derivative in your skin into vitamin D. In addition to its role in the maintenance of strong bones, vitamin D may also fight depression and possibly even help prevent cancer.

Vitamin E

Vitamin E is an antioxidant that can help your body avoid damage from free radicals, protect your cell membranes, and maintain heart health. Vitamin E aids in the production of red blood cells and assists your body in its usage of vitamin K. It may even act as a blood thinner, helping to lower your risk of blood clots.

Vitamin K

While *vitamin K* is mainly known for its role in helping your blood to clot properly, it has also been associated with bone health. Vitamin K helps your body use calcium to build bone. In fact, studies have suggested a link between low levels of vitamin K and osteoporosis. Evidence also points to the idea that vitamin K reduces your risk of bone fracture.

Vitamin K deficiency is a rare phenomenon, as the bacteria in your intestines are able to produce vitamin K. Taking antibiotics can kill bacteria in your digestive tract and lead to a deficiency, but you would have to have fairly low levels of this vitamin to begin with. Vitamin K deficiency may result in excessive bleeding.

■ MINERALS

Minerals account for approximately 4 to 5 percent of your body weight. Similar to vitamins, minerals play a role in many biological reactions, including the transmission of messages through your nervous system, muscle response, digestion and metabolism, and hormone production. Also similar to vitamins, minerals are micronutrients that are generally acquired from food in order to maintain sufficient amounts in your blood. Minerals are crucial to your bone development, brain health, cellular function, and metabolism. *Major minerals,* such as calcium, potassium, sodium, magnesium, are required in larger amounts than are minerals such as copper, iodine, iron, manganese, selenium, and zinc, which are considered *trace minerals.*

Calcium and Phosphorus

Calcium and *phosphorus* are *electrolytes*, meaning that they create an electrically conducting solution when dissolved in your body, enabling them to carry a charge. They are necessary for normal muscle and nerve activity, and are also crucial to the formation of bones and teeth and proper blood clotting. Adequate calcium, along with regular exercise and a healthy diet, helps regulate blood pressure, maintain good bone health, and reduce the chances of teen and young adult females getting osteoporosis later in their lives.

Choline

Choline is necessary component in the process by which your body carries cholesterol from your liver. As such, it prevents fat and cholesterol from building up in your liver. Choline also plays a role in brain development, DNA synthesis, and cell messaging, and is required an important *neurotransmitter*, or chemical messenger, called acetylcholine, which is involved in muscle movement, heart-beat regulation, and memory.

Chromium

Chromium helps remove sugar from your bloodstream and convert it into energy, which makes it a beneficial nutrient to individuals with type 2 diabetes. Chromium is necessary in the formation of *glucose tolerance factor* (GTF), a complex that works with the hormone insulin to maintain healthy blood glucose levels.

Copper

Along with iron, *copper* is a necessary component in the formation of red blood cells and nerve fibers. It is also a required element in the formation of the hair and skin pigment known as *melanin*. Copper is also known to have anti-inflammatory properties, help combat arthritis, and stimulate your brain.

Iodine

Iodine is an essential component of thyroid hormones, which regulate your metabolic rate. It aids in your body's metabolism of fat, helps in energy production and growth, and is vital to proper fetal development.

Iron

Iron helps in the transport of oxygen from your lungs to the rest of your body by being a necessary component of the protein hemoglobin in your blood. It is also part of the protein myoglobin, which makes oxygen available for muscle contractions. As previously noted, anemia refers to a lack of iron in your blood, and is a condition associated with weakness and low energy.

Magnesium

Magnesium is an electrolyte that plays an important role in your heart function (it helps your heart maintain a normal rhythm) and nervous system function. It also participates in the formation of your bones and teeth, aids in your body's conversion of glucose into energy, helps your blood to clot, and is required for calcium and vitamin C metabolism.

Manganese

Manganese improves your bone density, fights free radicals, helps regulate your blood sugar, and plays a part in the metabolism of the macronutrients protein, carbohydrates, and fat. It also aids in the formation of connective tissue, absorption of calcium, thyroid health, and sex hormone function.

Potassium, Sodium, and Chloride

Potassium, sodium, and *chloride* are electrolytes that maintain water levels in your bloodstream and thus help control your blood pressure. The electrical charges they carry aid in the transmission of nerve impulses and muscle contraction. These minerals are easily lost through sweat. Once they have been lost, they must then be replenished through your diet. Sodium and chloride are typically acquired in the form of sodium chloride, or salt. While eating too much salt, which is a very common problem in the modern world, may increase your risk of heart disease, potassium consumption can counteract this negative effect of sodium chloride.

Selenium

Selenium is a trace mineral that encourages healthy cognitive function, immune system function, and fertility in men and women. It is involved in thyroid hormone metabolism and DNA synthesis. It has attracted considerable attention for its role as a constituent of the antioxidant enzyme *glutathione peroxidase,* which may be found in your red blood cells and helps detoxify the byproducts of oxidized fat.

Zinc

Zinc is a mineral that is associated with many important functions in your body, although only a small amount is necessary in your diet. Zinc aids in the activity of over 100 different enzymes in every organ of your body. It regulates the way in which your neurons communicate with each other, affects how your memories are formed, helps manage insulin and thus plays a role in blood sugar control, is involved in the manufacture of genetic material and proteins, assists in the transport of vitamin A, and encourages proper taste perception, wound healing, cardiovascular health, sperm production, brain function, and fetal development. It also helps activate *T lymphocytes* in your body, which are cells that control and regulate your immune responses and attack infected or cancerous cells.

CONCLUSION

Your body requires a wide variety of nutrients in order to function optimally. The six major nutrients—carbohydrates, fat, protein, vitamins, minerals, and water—provide your body with energy, promote cell growth, assist in proper organ function, and maintain the health of your immune system. They help keep your blood and circulation in good working order, and your blood reciprocates by transporting these nutrients to the areas of your body that need them, aiding in the elimination of certain unwanted byproducts of nutrient metabolism, and generally keeping you alive and well every day. Once you understand the ways in which macronutrients and micronutrients impact your well-being, you gain a greater appreciation for the importance of diet and a more critical eye towards your choices at meal times.

5

Choosing Your Food

Arguably, the foods you choose to eat each day have the greatest impact on your blood, and thus on your health and well-being, of virtually any other aspect of your normal routine. Simply put, good food choices promote good health while bad food choices promote ill health. Although lifestyle and genetics also affect your risk of illness, of the ten leading causes of death in the United States, four of them have established connections to diet. These include the top three causes of death—heart disease, cancer, and stroke—as well as type 2 diabetes. Taken together, these four conditions account for 60 percent of the nation's more than 2 million deaths each year. Similar statistics can be found worldwide, with developing nations beginning to reflect many of the same levels of chronic diseases as developed nations.[1]

FOOD AND FOUR MAJOR ILLNESSES

There are a few nutritional risk factors that are common to two or more of these four chronic diseases, including a diet high in saturated fat or trans fat, excessive alcohol intake, low fiber intake, and low vitamin or mineral intake. This part of the chapter takes a closer look at the numerous well-researched links between food and these four conditions.

Heart Disease

Heart disease is usually caused by atherosclerosis in your coronary arteries, which supply blood to your heart muscle. As discussed in Chapter 2, atherosclerosis is the narrowing of arteries due to an accumulation of cholesterol and other lipids and materials, also known as plaque, in these blood vessels. When plaque narrows the internal diameter of a coronary artery enough to restrict blood flow and deprive your heart muscle of oxygen, heart disease develops. If you suffer from heart disease, you experience pain and pressure in the area around your heart, also known as angina. If blood flow to your heart is significantly reduced or cut off, your heart will not receive the oxygen it needs to survive, resulting in a heart attack.

A diet that promotes atherosclerosis is called an *atherogenic diet.* It elevates dangerous LDL cholesterol by being high in saturated fat, trans fat, and cholesterol, and low in fruits and vegetables. Conversely, a diet rich in fruits, vegetables, and whole grains has been shown to lower your risk of heart disease. This may be due to the consumption of specific nutrients in this type of diet, including omega-3 fatty acids and other antioxidants.[2]

Note that whole grains, not refined grains, contribute toward the reduced risk of heart disease. One reason for this distinction is that whole grains (as well as vegetables and fruits) are high in soluble fiber, and soluble fiber helps reduce your body's absorption of cholesterol, which might otherwise contribute to plaque buildup in your arteries.[3]

Research has shown that the highly processed, calorie-dense, nutrient-depleted diet favored in the current American culture frequently leads to dramatic spikes in blood sugar and blood fat levels after meals.[4] These spikes induce oxidative stress, which increases in direct proportion to the elevations in blood sugar and fat after a meal. This result triggers atherogenic changes in your body, including inflammation, dysfunction of the lining of your blood vessels, hypercoagulability (i.e., "sludgy blood"), and nervous system hyperactivity. These spikes may be viewed as independent predictors of future cardiovascular events. The good news is that you can reduce them by improving your diet.

Specifically, a diet high in minimally processed, high-fiber plant-based food, such as vegetables, fruits, whole grains, legumes, and nuts, will markedly lower your post-meal increases in blood sugar and fat, and therefore help you avoid their associated harmful atherogenic effects on your blood vessels. Experimental and epidemiological studies indicate that eating patterns such as the traditional Mediterranean diet or Okinawan diet, which incorporate these foods, reduce inflammation and cardiovascular risk. Thus, an anti-inflammatory diet should be considered for the primary and secondary prevention of heart disease as well as type 2 diabetes.[5]

Cancer

Cancer involves the growth of malignant tissue. There are many forms of cancer, or more specifically, many types of malignant growths. These cancers have different characteristics, occur in different locations in the body, develop differently, and require different treatments.

Cancer arises from mutations in the genes that control cell division in a single cell. These mutations may promote cellular growth or prevent cellular death. The affected cell then loses its natural ability to halt cell division and produces daughter cells with the same genetic defects. This abnormal mass of cells, or tumor, grows and can disrupt the functioning of the normal tissue around it. Some tumor cells metastasize, or spread to one or more regions in the body.

There are various reasons that cancers develop, including genetic, environmental, lifestyle, and dietary factors. These factors may alter cellular DNA structure, function, or repair, resulting in the mutations discussed previously. Regarding diet, as many as one-third of all cancers may be related to diet. In addition, certain chemicals used in our food supply may also contribute to cancer risk. For example, some pesticides are carcinogenic at high doses (although these can be largely avoided by consuming a diet consisting mainly of organic food).

Research has consistently shown that those with a high intake of whole grains have a lower risk of several types of cancer compared with those who consume few whole grains. These cancer types include cancers of the oral cavity, pharynx, larynx, esophagus, colorectum, stomach, liver, gallbladder, breast, ovary, prostate, bladder, kidney, and thyroid, as well as non-Hodgkin's lymphoma.[6,7] Again, the evidence here is for whole grains, not refined grains.

A panel of experts from the World Cancer Research Fund and the American Institute for Cancer Research reviewed research from hundreds of studies to determine the effects of food, nutrition, and physical activity on the prevention of cancer. In regard to vegetables and fruits, the results of their research were as follows:[8]

- Non-starchy vegetables, such as broccoli, Brussels sprouts, and cabbage, offer varying degrees of protection against cancers of the mouth, nasopharnx, pharynx, larynx, esophagus, stomach, lung, colorectum, ovary, and endometrium.

- Vegetables in the *Allium* genus, such as garlic and onions, offer protection against stomach and colorectal cancer.

- Carrots may protect against cervical cancer.

- Legumes, including soy and soy products, protect against stomach and prostate cancers.

- Many types of fruit protect against cancers of the mouth, pharynx, larynx, esophagus, lung, and stomach, and may also protect against cancers of the nasopharynx, pancreas, liver, and colorectum.

Families of fruits and vegetables share components that may offer particular health benefits. For example, cruciferous vegetables (e.g., broccoli, cauliflower, cabbage, Brussels sprouts, bok choy, and kale) are sources of glucosinolates and their metabolites, isothiocyanates and indoles. These compounds have been linked to a reduction in cancer risk, most strongly in connection with cancers of the mouth, pharynx, larynx, esophagus, and stomach.[9]

Stroke

Stroke has essentially the same causes as heart disease, but in the case of stroke, blood flow is restricted to your brain instead of your heart. Likewise, a diet rich in fruits, vegetables, and whole grains (not refined grains) lowers your risk of stroke just as it does your risk of heart attack.[12] In fact, research has shown that stroke risk can be significantly reduced through the use of a Mediterranean diet.[13] (See page 107.)

Generally, healthy diets include fruits, vegetables, fish, and whole grains, while limiting unhealthy fat. Subtle variations in the proportions of certain foods in healthy diets may make a difference in your risks of stroke and heart disease. This notion is particularly true of the Mediterranean diet. According to the Mayo Clinic, key aspects of the Mediterranean diet include:[14]

- Eating a generous amount of fruits and vegetables.

- Consuming healthy fats, such as those found in olive oil and canola oil.

- Eating small portions of nuts.

- Drinking red wine in moderation, for some.

- Consuming very little red meat.

- Eating fish on a regular basis.

As an example of the Mediterranean diet, residents of Greece eat very little red meat and eat about nine servings of antioxidant-rich fruits and vegetables daily. This type of eating has been associated with lowering levels of oxidized LDL cholesterol in your blood, which is more likely than other types of cholesterol to build up and form deposits in your arteries. Furthermore, grains in the Mediterranean region are typically whole grain and usually contain very few unhealthy fats.[15]

Diabetes

Epidemiological studies have shown that a high intake of carbo-hydrates from refined grains and potatoes is associated with an increase in risks of type 2 diabetes and coronary heart disease.[16] Consumption of whole grains was not similarly implicated in these studies. Why is this the case? The answer probably has to do with the glycemic index (GI).

The glycemic index is a numerical system of measuring how fast a carbohydrate triggers a rise in circulating blood sugar—the higher the number, the higher the elevation of your blood sugar. So, a low GI food will cause a small rise, while a high GI food will trigger a dramatic spike. Consistent, dramatic spikes in your blood sugar are more likely to increase your risk of diabetes. The glycemic effect of a food may be greatly influenced by its fiber content. For example, high-fiber grain-based foods are more likely to be lower on the glycemic index than those made with refined grains, which are low in fiber. Fiber causes a food to break down more slowly in your digestive system, thus reducing the rate of absorption of any sugars it contains. The result is a slower increase in your blood glucose level. By contrast, products made with refined grains, such white bread and white pasta, break down rapidly and yield their sugars quickly, spiking your blood glucose level.

The GI number of a food is also influenced by preparation method (see page 101) and the other foods included in your meal.[17] As with heart disease, a diet high in minimally processed, high-fi-ber plant-based foods, such as vegetables, fruit, whole grains, legumes, and nuts, reduces post-meal increases in blood sugar and fats, as well as inflammation, and thus may help prevent type

2 diabetes.[18] This idea has been validated by population studies that show an association between high-GI diets and a rise in type 2 diabetes risk. Conversely, the available evidence suggests that eating a diet rich in vegetables and whole grains and low in refined grains, sucrose, and fructose is beneficial in the prevention of type 2 diabetes.[19]

■ GRAINS

Grains, such as corn, barley, oats, rice, rye, and wheat, contain many healthful components, including fiber, B vitamins (thiamin, or B_1; riboflavin, or B_2; niacin, or B_3; and folate, or B_9) and minerals (iron, magnesium, and selenium). In addition to reducing spikes in your blood sugar levels, dietary fiber from whole grains also helps lower blood cholesterol levels and may decrease your risk of heart disease. Fiber is important for healthy bowel function and helps reduce constipation. B vitamins help your body release energy from protein, fat, and carbohydrates. Iron is used to carry oxygen in your blood. Magnesium is a mineral used in building bones and releasing energy from your muscles. Selenium is important for a healthy immune system. Three to eight ounces of grains are recommended each day, depending on how many calories you need.[20,21]

Whole Wheat Flour vs White Flour

In terms of the relationship between dietary grains and your health, whole grains are preferred over refined grains. To understand why this is the case, consider a kernel of wheat. The kernel is essentially made up of three major layers: 1) the bran, 2) the germ, and 3) the endosperm. Each of these layers provides certain nutrients, and each contributes to the total nutrition of the overall wheat kernel.

The bran layer is the outermost part of the grain. It contributes significant amounts of fiber, as well as minerals (iron, magnesium, phosphorus, potassium, zinc, copper, manganese, selenium) and even some vitamins (B_1, B_2, B_3, B_5, B_6).[22] The germ layer is the part of the grain that can sprout into a new plant. It contains many of the same vitamins and minerals found in the bran layer, in addition to excellent quantities of folate (vitamin B_9) and a respectable amount of protein.[23] The endosperm acts as a source of energy for the germ and is primarily a starchy carbohydrate with comparatively few minerals or vitamins.[24]

A 100-percent whole wheat food product will have been made using flour from ground wheat kernels with all three layers. This flour will thus contain all the naturally occurring nutrients of the complete grains. When wheat is refined however, the resultant flour is drastically different. Refined wheat flour (i.e., white flour) is made from grains that have had their bran and germ layers removed. Oftentimes refined flour is bleached to make it whiter, and to enhance the bonding qualities of its gluten protein.

Unfortunately, this refinement process reduces the protein level in the flour by about 19 percent, and decreases its dietary fiber amount by a whopping 80 percent. Furthermore, of the minerals and vitamins originally present, all levels are lowered substantially through refinement. In an inadequate attempt to compensate, iron and B vitamins are generally added to white flour at levels higher than originally present in a process referred to as "enrichment."

■ FRUIT

The term "fruit" normally means the fleshy seed-containing structures of a plant that are sweet or sour, and edible in their raw state, such as apples, bananas, grapes, lemons, oranges, and strawberries. Fruit is an important source of fiber and can offer a wide variety of nutrients, including potassium, vitamin C, and vitamin B_9, or folate. These nutrients are vital to the health and maintenance of your body. The potassium in fruit can reduce your risk of heart disease and stroke. Potassium may also reduce your risk of developing kidney stones and help decrease bone loss as you age. Folate helps your body form red blood cells. Women of childbearing age who may become pregnant and those in the first trimester of pregnancy need adequate folate intake. Folate helps prevent neural tube birth defects, such as spina bifida. Fruit such as blueberries, citrus fruit, cranberries, and strawberries also contain other compounds that are being studied for their health benefits.

Eating a diet rich in fruit may lower your chances of stroke, other cardiovascular diseases, and type 2 diabetes. Fruit consumption is part of an overall healthy diet and may protect against certain cancers. Finally, other chemical compounds produced by plants, also known as *phytochemicals,* are still being identified in fruit. Depending on your caloric needs, it is recommended that you eat 1 to 2 1/2 cups of fruit each day.[25,26]

■ VEGETABLES

People who eat fruit and vegetables as part of their daily diets reduce their risks of many chronic diseases. Vegetables are an important part of healthy eating and provide many healthful compounds, including potassium, fiber, folate, vitamins A, vitamin E, and vitamin C. Potassium may help to maintain healthy blood pressure. Dietary fiber from vegetables helps reduce blood cholesterol levels and may lower your risk of heart disease. As discussed in connection with fruit, folate helps your body form healthy red blood cells. Women of childbearing age who may become pregnant and those in the first trimester of pregnancy need adequate folate to reduce the risk of neural tube defects during fetal development. The nutrients in vegetables are vital to the health and maintenance of your body. As well, options like broccoli, spinach, tomatoes, and garlic offer additional health benefits, which is why many people consider them to be "superfoods."

Simply put, eating a diet rich in vegetables may reduce your risks of stroke, cancer, heart diseases, and type 2 diabetes. Dietary guidelines suggest that you try to eat 1 to 4 cups of vegetables each day.[27]

■ PROTEIN-RICH FOODS

Meat, poultry, fish, legumes, eggs, nuts, and seeds supply your blood with many nutrients and are an important part of healthy eating. These foods include not only proteins but also B vitamins (B_1, B_2, B_3, B_6, and B_{12}), vitamin E, magnesium, zinc, and iron. The proteins found in meat, beans, and nuts serve as building blocks for bones, muscles, cartilage, skin, and blood. They are also associated with many enzymes and hormones. B vitamins found in this food group aid in a variety of functions in your body. They help your body release energy and build tissue. Vitamin B_{12} is needed for healthy blood and, due to the fact that the plants we eat now are much cleaner and lack the presence of bacterial sources of vitamin B_{12}, this vitamin is found only in animal products.

If you follow a vegan diet—meaning that you don't eat any food derived from animal sources—you may need to take a supplement to get your vitamin B_{12}, although many vegan products are fortified with B_{12}. Nuts and seeds are excellent sources of healthful essential fatty acids and vitamin E. Depending on your caloric needs, aim to eat 46 g to 56 g of protein each day.[28]

Meat

In general, red meat (beef, pork, lamb) has more cholesterol and saturated fat than do other sources of protein, such as chicken, fish, or legumes. Cholesterol and saturated fat can raise your blood cholesterol and make heart disease worse. Chicken and fish have less saturated fat than most red meat. The unsaturated fats found in fish such as salmon actually have health benefits. Omega-3 fatty acids, which are available in fish and some plant sources, may reduce your risk of cardiovascular disease.

This is not to say that you should not eat red meat at all. You may do so as long as you limit the amount you consume. The American Heart Association recommends that people limit their total consumption of lean meat, skinless chicken, and fish to less than six ounces a day. Fish should be eaten at least twice a week, preferably fish high in omega-3 fatty acids, such as salmon, trout, and herring.[29] In order to keep your blood running smoothly, lower the amount of saturated fat and cholesterol you get when you eat meat by choosing lean cuts of meat. A lean cut of red meat usually features the word "round," "loin," or "sirloin" on its package. Trim off as much fat as you can before cooking and pour off the melted fat after cooking. Finally, opt for healthier cooking methods such as baking, broiling, stewing, or grilling.

Legumes

Foods known as legumes are actually the edible fruits or seeds, sometimes called pulses, of plants in the legume family. Examples of legumes include peas, beans, chickpeas, lentils, soybeans, and peanuts. Legumes are significant sources of protein, dietary fiber, carbohydrates, and minerals. For instance, 100 g of cooked chickpeas contains 18 percent of the recommended daily intake for protein, 30 percent for dietary fiber, 43 percent for folate, and 52 percent for manganese. Like other plant-based foods, legumes contain no cholesterol and little fat or sodium.[30] In addition, legumes are rich in resistant starch, which is broken down by bacteria in your large intestine to produce short-chain fatty acids that are then used by your intestinal cells as energy source.[31] Some also suggest that regular consumption of legumes in a vegetarian diet can help reduce the risk of metabolic syndrome, also known as prediabetes.[32]

Nuts and Seeds

While it is true that nuts and seeds are high in fat and calories, the fat they provide is heart-healthy unsaturated fat. They also contain protein, fiber, antioxidants, and substances known as *plant stanols,* which may help lower the level of LDL cholesterol in your blood. Research has found that including a serving of nuts (approximately a handful) in your diet may actually prevent weight gain and possibly even promote weight loss, as long as you control total calories. The protein, fiber, and fat in nuts aid in satiety and help you feel full longer, so you may actually end up eating less during the day. Nut eaters have also been shown to have a lower incidence of type 2 diabetes when compared to those who rarely eat nuts.[33]

■ DAIRY

A glass of milk contains three of the four nutrients that the United States Department of Agriculture (USDA) deems under-consumed by most Americans: calcium, vitamin D, and potassium. Thus, it is recommended that adults eat two servings of low-fat or fat-free dairy products each day. Dairy products are made from milk and include cheese, yogurt, and ice cream. The following portions are equal to one serving of dairy:

- 1 cup of 1-percent or skim milk

- 1 cup of low-fat or fat-free yogurt

- 2 ounces of low-fat or fat-free cheese

Low-fat or fat-free dairy can have just as much flavor and texture as dairy made with whole milk; it just has less saturated fat.[34] If you want to incorporate low-fat or fat-free dairy into your diet, have 1-percent or skim milk with your cereal, add sliced strawberries to your fat-free yogurt, make pizza with mozzarella cheese made with 1-percent or fat-free milk, add low-fat or fat-free feta cheese to your salad.

When most people think of milk, they think of its role in building strong bones. Your body uses many nutrients to encourage bone strength, and milk and other dairy foods provide a number of bone-building nutrients, specifically calcium, vitamin D, protein, phosphorus, magnesium, potassium, vitamin B_{12}, and zinc.

Finally, dairy is an important component of the DASH (Dietary Approaches to Stop Hypertension) diet, which is designed to reduce your risk of high blood pressure. This diet, which includes three servings a day of low-fat or fat-free milk, yogurt, or cheese, and eight to ten servings daily of fruits and vegetables, has also been shown to reduce your risk of heart disease and stroke.[35,36]

Lactose Intolerance

Not everyone, however, is able to consume dairy products without issue. Lactose, a sugar found in milk, is normally broken down by an enzyme called lactase, which is produced by cells in the lining of your small intestine. Some people have an impaired ability to digest lactose. This impairment is known as *lactose intolerance.*

Lactose intolerance in adulthood is caused by a reduction in the production of lactase after infancy, also known as *lactase nonpersistence.* If individuals with lactose intolerance consume lactose-containing dairy products, they may experience abdominal pain, bloating, flatulence, nausea, and diarrhea beginning thirty minutes to two hours later. Most people with lactase non-persistence retain some lactase activity and can include varying amounts of lactose in their diets without experiencing symptoms. Often, affected individuals have difficulty digesting fresh milk but can eat certain dairy products such as cheese or yogurt without discomfort. These foods are made using fermentation processes that break down much of the lactose in milk.

Individuals with lactose intolerance can chose to consume cow's milk with added lactase, or simply replace cow's milk with soy milk or almond milk.

■ WATER

Water is not only the most abundant nutrient found in the body (accounting for roughly 60 percent of adult body weight), but it is also involved in nearly every bodily function, including digestion, absorption, circulation, and excretion. Water provides no calories but is the primary transporter of nutrients throughout your body.

It participates in chemical reactions, acts as a solvent for vitamins, minerals, amino acids, and glucose, functions as a lubricant and cushion around joints, serves as a shock absorber in your eyes and spinal cord, and forms amniotic fluid to protect a growing fetus. Water helps maintain a normal body temperature and blood volume, while playing an essential role in carrying waste material out of your body.

How Much Water Do You Need?

Every day you lose water through your breath, perspiration, urine, and bowel movements. For your body to function properly, you must replenish its water supply by drinking water and consuming foods that contain water.

So, how much fluid does the average, healthy adult living in a temperate climate need? You've probably heard the advice, "Drink 8 eight-ounce glasses of water a day," but is this amount enough? According to the National Academies of Sciences, Engineering, and Medicine, an adequate daily fluid intake for me is about 15 1/2 cups of fluid a day, while an adequate intake for women is about 11 1/2 cups of fluid a day. These recommendations cover fluids from water, other beverages, and food. About 20 percent of daily fluid intake usually comes from food and the rest from drink.

■ HERBS AND SPICES

While the foods you eat can have significant effects on the health of your blood and thus your overall well-being, the herbs and spices you use to season your meals can also profoundly impact the state of your blood and body. For example, cinnamon is well known for its ability to lower your blood sugar, which it does by supporting insulin sensitivity. It also has significantly antioxidant potential. Ginger root has been recognized as a digestive aid and may also be considered a natural blood thinner, promoting healthy blood pressure. Turmeric, the spice that gives curry powder its distinctive yellow coloring, contains a compound called *curcumin,* which has anti-inflammatory and cancer-protective properties. It also promotes cardiovascular health by preventing blood clots, aiding in the regulation of blood pressure, and raising HDL cholesterol.

Hot peppers such as cayenne peppers contain a compound called *capsaicin,* which seems to provide cardiovascular benefits. In animal studies it has displayed the ability to relax blood vessels and lower blood pressure. Research has shown that rosemary can prevent the formation of chemicals known as *heterocyclic amines,* or HCAs, which typically occur when meat is cooked at high temperatures, and which can increase your risk of cancer. Rosemary has the potential to halt tumor development and stop carcinogens from binding to your DNA.

Coriander, also known as cilantro, is high in beta-carotene and can lower your risk of cardiovascular events as well as prostate cancer. It can boost your immune system and is known as a detoxifying agent that helps eliminate mercury from your body. Finally, basil helps your liver and kidneys remove unwanted material from your body. It also acts as a diuretic, encouraging the production of urine in your body, thus further helping remove any harmful substances that may be circulating in your blood.

Of course, in addition to the previous examples, many other herbs and spices offer health benefits, and you should continue to try new seasoning options as much as you can.

COOKING TECHNIQUES

As you may already know, it is not only your choice of food that can impact the health of your blood and body but also the way in which you prepare your food. Cooking techniques account for many of the reasons why a particular meal might have a positive or negative effect on your well-being.

Perhaps the most well-known example of this idea is the way in which cooking can lead to a loss of nutrients in vegetables and fruit. Water-soluble vitamins, which include vitamins B and C, are the most easily depleted through cooking, while the content of fat-soluble vitamins, which include vitamins A, D, and E, does not suffer as much from the process. Although boiling or steaming is better than frying when it comes to the maintaining the nutrient contents of vegetables, microwaving often preserves the most nutrients in food.

While you might assume that raw vegetables and fruit are your best choice in terms of vitamin and mineral contents, sometimes the process of cooking actually increases amounts of certain healthful substances in these foods, breaking down the thick cellular walls of many plants and thereby releasing their nutrients. For example, a cooked tomato will have a much higher lycopene content than will a raw tomato.

Food preparation influences a food's glycemic index number as well. Cooking in general tends to raise the glycemic index value of a food simply by making that food more easily digestible. For example, the longer you boil pasta, the higher its glycemic index number will be. In addition, boiling carrots more than doubles their GI value. Adding fat, fiber, or an acidic component, such as lemon juice or vinegar, to your meal, however, lowers that meals glycemic index.

As previously mentioned in this chapter, cooking meat at high heat promotes the formation of harmful chemicals called heterocyclic amines, or HCAs. In addition, cooking meat over an open fire or smoking meat creates dangerous compounds known as *polycyclic aromatic hydrocarbons,* or PAHs. These substances cause inflammation in your body and have been linked to cancer. Stewing or steaming meat results in the creation of fewer HCAs, and, as you now know, cooking with rosemary also inhibits HCA formation. For those who still wish to smoke meat or cook it over an open flame, marinating the meat in acidic ingredients, such as lemon juice or vinegar, has been shown to cut the formation of PAHs significantly.

SOURCES OF MICRONUTRIENTS

Micronutrients may be found in supplements of all kinds, which can help fill in gaps in your diet and prevent deficiencies. Getting vitamins and minerals the old-fashioned way, though, through real food instead of supplements, is best, as doing so helps your body to absorb and utilize them properly. In fact, studies have shown that the complex mixture of micronutrients found naturally in a diet high in fruit and vegetables is likely to be more effective in terms of promoting good health than are large doses of a small number of micronutrients.

Vary your diet and include lots of colorful foods in your meals, especially vegetables and fruits, which are high in vitamins, minerals, and antioxidants. By using many different foods in your daily menu, you are sure to consume a range of macronutrients—healthy fats, carbs, and proteins—as well.

Here are a few specific foods that supply high levels of multiple micronutrients:

Fruit (Especially Berries): Strawberries, blueberries, raspberries, melon, pineapple, apples, pears and kiwis are high in antioxidants such as flavanoids, vitamins A and C, potassium, fiber. Berries, in particular, are associated with brain health and cancer prevention. They have high ORAC (Oxygen Radical Absorption Capacity) scores, a measurement that determines the power of a food to absorb and eliminate free radicals. Many berries, including blueberries, are high in quercetin, a type of protective flavonoid phytonutrient that fights inflammation.

Leafy Green Vegetables: All kinds of greens are excellent sources of vitamin C, vitamin A, vitamin K, folate, and magnesium. Considering how low in calories leafy greens like kale, collard greens, spinach, bok choy, cabbage, and romaine lettuce are, they're some of the most nutrient-dense foods available.

Other Colorful Vegetables: Red peppers, broccoli, squash, cauliflower, green peppers, artichokes, carrots, asparagus, tomatoes, and mushrooms are all great sources of magnesium, potassium, vitamin A, vitamin C, and fiber. Basically, all vegetables provide micronutrients in moderate to high levels, so during meals try filling half your plate with a mix of veggies as often as you can.

Legumes: Some of the best sources of fiber, beans are great for digestion and controlling cholesterol. They're also high in calcium, manganese, folate, phosphorus, and iron.

Nuts and Seeds: Omega-3 fatty acids and high levels of fiber are some of the benefits that come with eating nuts and seeds such as chia, flax, hemp, almonds, and walnuts. Nuts and seeds are also great sources of antioxidants like vitamin E, and micronutrients such as selenium, magnesium, boron, and choline.

Grass-fed/Pasture-Raised/Wild Animal Products: Liver, wild seafood, cage-free eggs, grass-fed beef, and pasture-raised poultry are excellent sources of micronutrients such as iron, B vitamins, vitamin A, and zinc. Each type of animal protein offers different benefits. For example, chicken or beef liver is packed with micronutrients. In fact, it is now being called a "superfood" because it is rich in B vitamins, iron, and vitamin A. Finally, cage-free eggs offer multiple nutrients, including choline, vitamin A, and vitamin E.

Whole Grains: Ancient grains like quinoa, rice, amaranth, oats, and buckwheat provide B vitamins, as well as minerals such as manganese and phosphorus. While ancient grains can be a part of a balanced diet, I recommend getting even higher levels of micronutrients and dietary fiber from more nutrient-dense foods like non-starchy veggies, starchy veggies, and fruit.

GOING ORGANIC

Whenever possible, do your best to choose food that has been organically grown. But what does the designation "organic" actually mean in regard to food? The USDA website answers this question by stating:

Organic food is produced by farmers who emphasize the use of renewable resources and the conservation of soil and water to enhance environmental quality for future generations. Organic meat, poultry, eggs, and dairy products come from animals that are given no antibiotics or growth hormones. Organic food is produced without using most conventional pesticides; fertilizers made with synthetic ingredients or sewage sludge; bioengineering; or ionizing radiation. Before a product can be labeled "organic," a Government-approved certifier inspects the farm where the food is grown to make sure the farmer is following all the rules necessary to meet USDA organic standards. Companies that handle or process organic food before it gets to your local supermarket or restaurant must be certified, too.[37]

Organically grown food offers Americans a healthier alternative to conventionally grown food. Let us examine the evidence. In 2002, Dr. Erik Steen Kristensen of the Danish Research Centre for Organic Farming presented data on food safety from an organic perspective at the 14th International Federation of Organic Agriculture Movements Congress in Victoria, Canada.[38] Dr. Kristensen offered a number of reasons to consider organic foods, including the discovery of animals with bovine spongiform encephalopathy (BSE), also known as mad cow disease. This neurodegenerative disease is fatal in cattle and transmissible to humans who have consumed infected meat. Investigations have shown that animals contract this disease by eating ground up animal byproducts in their feed. Organic meat, however, does not come from animals that have been fed animal byproducts.

Another reason to opt for organic food is the high amounts of pesticides, antibiotics, and additives associated with nonorganic choices. As well, various data indicate that compared with conventionally grown produce, organically grown produce has higher vitamin C levels,[39,40] lower nitrate levels (less carcinogenic potential),[41] higher phenol levels (protection against cancer and cardiovascular disease),[42] lower levels of heavy metals,[43] lower or zero levels of food additives (less food intolerance and carcinogenic potential).[44] Likewise, research shows that compared with conventional animal foods, organic animal foods have higher levels of conjugated linoleic acid or CLA (preventive against cancer and arteriosclerosis),[45] higher levels of vitamin C,[46] higher levels of fat-soluble vitamins,[47] higher levels of omega-3 fatty acids,[48] zero mycotoxins (less potential problems for your liver, kidney, and nervous system),[49] lower levels of medicinal residues.[50] Studies show higher fertility and lower morbidity rates in animals given organic feed.[51,52]

Collectively, these findings make a pretty good case for choosing to eat organic food whenever you can.

THE IMPACT OF POPULAR DIETS ON HEALTH

When discussing the impact food can have on your blood and health, it is reasonable to detail a few of the most popular diets and their effects. The following section outlines the low-carb/high-protein diet, the Mediterranean diet, the "MyPlate" diet, and the plant-based diet.

Low-Carb/High-Protein Diet

The low-carb/high-protein diet was made popular by the late Dr. Robert Atkins. In fact, it is often referred to as the Atkins diet. In addition to its low carbohydrate and high protein profile, the diet plan is also relatively high in fat. Part of the rationale for the lower consumption of carbohydrates is so that too much glucose, or sugar, does not tax your body's metabolism. In essence, Dr. Atkins proposed that the body regularly produces insulin to convert excess carbohydrates into body fat, and so excess carbohydrates must be eliminated so as not to create more fat.[53] While a number of scientific studies using the low-carbohydrate diet lend support to this approach for successful weight loss,[54,55] the high saturated-fat content of this diet may make it a bad idea for anyone who is at high risk for heart disease.

Mediterranean Diet

The Mediterranean diet is based upon the diets of at least sixteen countries that border the Mediterranean Sea. Although there are many differences in culture, ethnic background, religion, economy, and agricultural production, which result in variations in food intake among these population groups, there is still a common Mediterranean dietary pattern that includes: 1) high consumption of fruits, vegetables, bread and other whole grain cereals, potatoes, beans, nuts, and seeds; 2) olive oil as an important monounsaturated fat source; 3) dairy products, fish, and poultry consumed in low to moderate amounts, with little red meat eaten; 4) eggs consumed zero to four times a week; and 5) wine consumed in low to moderate amounts. Consequently, this diet tends to be low on the GI, with a good balance of dietary fats. Research has shown that the Mediterranean diet reduces mortality rates and rates of fatal and nonfatal heart attack, and provides protection against coronary heath disease.[56,57] Furthermore, the Mediterranean diet has been shown to promote good control of blood glucose levels.[58]

MyPlate Diet

The USDA's "MyPlate" diet plan is meant to provide Americans with the ability to personalize their approaches when choosing a healthier lifestyle that balances nutrition and exercise. At the same time, MyPlate is not "a therapeutic diet for any specific health condition,"[59] although recommendations in MyPlate are remarkably consistent with the various methods to control obesity and diabetes, heart disease and stroke, hypertension, cancer, and osteoporosis that have been suggested by the American Diabetes Association, the National Cholesterol Education Program, the American Heart Association, and the National Committee on High Blood Pressure.

Plant-Based Diet

Although not always easy to follow, a raw vegan diet contains fewer foods that elicit an increase in blood glucose and insulin levels than do most other ways of eating.[60] Results of this diet may be seen in case reports that indicate that diabetic patients who were placed on a diet containing an increased percentage of raw vegan food were able to decrease their insulin requirements. In fact, one patient had his insulin requirement reduced from 60 units per day to 15 units per day. Furthermore, long-term consumption of a low-calorie, low-protein vegan diet is associated with low cardiovascular disease risk.[61] This includes lower body mass index (BMI), lower plasma concentrations of lipids, lipoproteins, glucose, insulin, and C-reactive protein, as well as lower blood pressure (both systolic and diastolic). Long-term benefits have also been seen in a seventeen-year observational study of vegetarians and other health-conscious people. Results demonstrated that daily consumption of fresh fruit was associated with significantly reduced mortality from ischemic heart disease and cerebrovascular disease, and for all causes combined.[62] Overall, the individuals in the study had a mortality about half that of the general population. In addition, in a twelve-week study, individuals following a raw food vegan diet experienced improvement in measurements of mental and emotional quality of life.[63]

CONCLUSION

Compared with virtually any other aspect of your daily life, the foods you choose to eat can have the single greatest impact on your blood and overall well-being. Of the ten leading causes of death in the United States, four of them (heart disease, cancer, stroke, and type 2 diabetes) have a relationship with diet. An optimal diet to help promote and maintain good health includes a daily balance between whole grains, fruit, vegetables, protein-rich food, low-fat or fat-free dairy, and water.

6

Oxygen
and Your Blood

Although food, liquid, and oxygen are all required for your body's survival, oxygen has a special role in this process, as it is the compound that allows your cells to produce energy from the foods and liquids you ingest. Without oxygen, your body could not use these substances as fuel to generate the power it needs to sustain itself. Specifically, through a mechanism known as oxidation, oxygen chemically changes food and liquid into energy for use by your body. It is oxygen that is responsible for muscle contractions, brain function, and calming your nerves. It even helps repair your cells.

When these processes happen, carbon dioxide is produced as a waste product. Just as your lungs take in oxygen from the environment and provide it to your blood, so do they allow your body to get rid of this waste gas. In fact, your body constantly sends signals to your brain that tell it the levels of oxygen and carbon dioxide in your blood. Based on this information, your brain tells your muscles to adjust your breathing rate appropriately, increasing it to prevent a buildup of carbon dioxide in your bloodstream when necessary.

This chapter will discuss how important oxygen is to your health and wellness in relation to its presence in your blood. First, let us review how your blood actually goes about transporting oxygen throughout your body.

THE TRANSPORTATION OF OXYGEN

Oxygen is transported throughout your body by your blood. As previously described, your blood contains plasma, which comprises red blood cells, white blood cells, and platelets. It is your red blood cells that are crucial to the transportation of oxygen. Red blood cells are formed in your bone marrow and contain hemoglobin, which is what give them their color. Hemoglobin is also responsible for carrying oxygen. Oxygen molecules attach themselves to the hemoglobin in your blood as it travels through your lungs, where the oxygen you breathe passes through thin capillary walls into your bloodstream.

Once oxygen has attached itself to hemoglobin, your oxygenated blood is moved from your lungs to your heart, which then pumps this blood through your arteries, which send it throughout your body. This oxygenated blood delivers oxygen to the tissues in need of it. Deoxygenated blood is then brought back to your lungs to pick up more fresh oxygen. The carbon dioxide waste gas that has hitched a ride to your lungs during this process is expelled at this time as you exhale.

Hemoglobin also transports nitric oxide, a compound created by your body that opens up your blood vessels. This widening of your blood vessels is known as a *vasodilatory effect*. Dilation of your blood vessels improves your circulation, thus assisting in the transportation and delivery of oxygen to your tissues.[1]

THE IMPORTANCE OF OXYGEN

Although many chemical elements are found in the human body, six of them are the most abundant and together account for more than 98 percent of body weight. They are oxygen, carbon, hydrogen, nitrogen, calcium, and phosphorus. Oxygen alone, in fact, is the most prevalent element, comprising 61 percent of body weight.[2] Human beings are able to survive for a few weeks without food, and for a few days without water; but without oxygen, humans last only a few minutes.

THE DARK SIDE OF OXYGEN

When your cells use oxygen to generate energy, free radicals are created as a result of the production of ATP by the *mitochondria*, which are the main producers of chemical energy in cells. These free radicals include reactive oxygen species (ROS) and reactive nitrogen species (RNS), which, at high concentrations, produce oxidative stress—a harmful process that can damage all cell structures.[3] Research suggests that most of the degenerative diseases currently afflicting humanity have their origins in the damage caused by free radicals.[4,5] These diseases include cardiovascular and neurodegenerative diseases, cancer, inflammatory joint disease, asthma, type 2 diabetes, dementia, degenerative eye disease, autoimmune disorders, and even aging. This is why it is so important to consume sufficient amounts of antioxidants, which are commonly found in fruit and vegetables, and which help reduce the effects of free radicals and diminish the oxidative stress they can cause.

As mentioned earlier, oxygen plays a critical role in turning the food and liquid you consume into energy. As explained in Chapter 4, the carbohydrates, fatty acids, and proteins in food are gradually broken down by your body and then oxidized in your cells. This metabolic process results in the release of energy from these macronutrients and the generation of ATP molecules (which trap this energy and help transfer it to your cells), carbon dioxide, and water. None of this could occur without oxygen.

Of course, oxygen performs another vital role in your body by being a component of the water molecule: H_2O. Your cells are about 70- to 90-percent water by mass, and without water and its ability to form hydrogen bonds, life would likely not be possible at all. It is due to the very high water content of cells that the human body is mostly oxygen. Needless to say, oxygen plays many, many important roles in your body.

HYPOXEMIA AND HYPOXIA

Low levels of oxygen in your blood result in a state known as *hypoxemia*. Low levels of oxygen in the tissues of your body lead to a state known as *hypoxia*. While hypoxemia can lead to hypoxia, hypoxia may also occur as a result of conditions that restrict the delivery of the oxygen in your blood to particular parts of your body.

Although all organs require oxygen, the brain and heart are particularly sensitive to a shortage of oxygen. As previously mentioned, a significant lack of oxygen that lasts only a few minutes can be fatal. Low levels of oxygen in the body have a number of possible causes, such as elevated altitude, respiratory ailments, pH level, anemia, fatigue, stress, and metabolic diseases, each of which may be categorized under a general subtype of hypoxia.[6]

Hypoxemic Hypoxia

Hypoxemic hypoxia is a subtype of hypoxia caused by a deficiency in the content of oxygen in your arterial blood. (As recently mentioned, a low level of oxygen in your blood is known as hypoxemia.) This deficiency occurs when there is a reduction in the amount of oxygen getting into your lungs. When there is less oxygen entering your lungs, there is less oxygen being transferred from your lungs into your blood. This condition may result from respiratory ailments such as asthma or pneumonia, drowning, or the decreased oxygen levels in the air at high altitudes.

Altitude, in fact, can have a pronounced effect on your blood's oxygen uptake. Your blood's oxygen uptake reading may be 98 percent when you are at sea level, but as soon as you move up to 5,000 feet above sea level, it may drop to 95 percent. At 10,000 feet, it could be 90 percent. Mild hypoxemia sets in when your blood's oxygen uptake is between 90 and 94 percent. When you reach over 10,000 feet above sea level, you may not be able to adjust to the lack of oxygen, and your blood's oxygen uptake percentage may drop to dangerous numbers. Moderate hypoxemia occurs when your blood's oxygen uptake readings fall between 75 and 89 percent, while severe hypoxemia is any reading below 75 percent. Severe hypoxemia may lead to loss of consciousness and even brain damage.

Furthermore, there are factors that can affect your body's response to changes in altitude. These factors include medications such as aspirin, nitrites, and sulfa; diet; level of physical fitness; emotional state; chronic obstructive pulmonary disease (COPD); baseline metabolic rate; fever or low body temperature; and blood pH level (which refers to the acid-alkaline balance of your blood).

A low pH (acidic) makes it harder for the hemoglobin in your blood to bind to oxygen but easier for it to release bound oxygen to your tissues. Conversely, a high pH (alkaline) makes it easier for the hemoglobin to pick up oxygen but harder for it to release it to your tissues.[7]

PHYSIOLOGIC ALTITUDE

Some factors unrelated to atmospheric pressure can actually cause certain people to react as though they were at higher altitude even when they are at sea level. They can create what is known as a person's *physiologic altitude* and include the following:[8]

• **Smoking.** Smoking three cigarettes quickly or one to one and a half packs in one day at an average pace can create a physiological altitude of 2,000 feet.

• **Alcohol consumption.** Consuming one ounce of alcohol can create a physiological altitude of 2,000 feet.

• **Coffee consumption.** Drinking five cups of coffee can create a physiological altitude of 2,500 feet.

In other words, sometimes you don't have to climb a mountain to feel like you are halfway up one.

Anemic Hypoxia

In *anemic hypoxia* your lungs are able to take in sufficient amounts of oxygen, but your blood's ability to carry or deliver oxygen has been reduced. Your tissues, in turn, do not receive enough oxygen because your blood cannot bring it to them as effectively. As the its name suggests, this form of hypoxia may be caused by *anemia*, which is a deficiency in red blood cells, hemoglobin, or your blood's ability to carry oxygen. Anemia typically occurs due to a lack of iron in your blood, which usually results from poor iron intake, poor absorption of iron from food, or blood loss.

Carbon monoxide poisoning can also lead to anemic hypoxia. While the hemoglobin in your blood is responsible for binding to and transporting oxygen throughout your body, its affinity to bind to carbon monoxide is several hundred times greater than its affinity to bind to oxygen. Consequently, hemoglobin in blood will become saturated at much lower levels of carbon monoxide than of oxygen. For example, 50-percent saturation of hemoglobin may be achieved in the presence of carbon monoxide in an amount several hundred times less than the required amount of oxygen that would yield similar hemoglobin saturation. Thus, even very low levels of carbon monoxide in the air can have profound effects on the amount of oxygen available to your tissues.[9]

Conversely, in a condition known as *methemoglobinemia,* your red blood cells have plenty of oxygen but their ability to release it to the rest of your body's cells is impaired, thus leading to anemic hypoxia. Finally, anemic hypoxia may also result from the use of medications such as aspirin, sulfonamides, or nitrites.

Stagnant Hypoxia

In *stagnant hypoxia* your blood has a sufficient content of oxygen and is able to carry it properly but the flow of blood throughout your body is hampered. Poor blood flow may be the result of a number of issues, including heart failure, decreased circulating blood volume, pooling of blood in your veins due to gravitational forces, or g-forces, and poor vasodilation.

Vasodilation refers to the increase in the internal diameter of your blood vessels, or the widening of your blood vessels, which is caused by the relaxation of smooth muscle cells within the walls of these vessels, particularly in large arteries, small arterioles, and large veins. This widening of your blood vessels leads to an increase in blood flow. In fact, the primary function of vasodilation is to increase the flow of blood in your body, especially to the tissues where it is required most. This dilation happens most commonly when your tissues are in need of oxygen.[10] If vasodilation is poor or inadequate, blood flow slows down, as does delivery of oxygen to your tissues.

Histotoxic Hypoxia

Histotoxic hypoxia, or *histologic hypoxia,* differs from the others because it does not involve any problem in getting oxygen to tissues via your lungs, blood, and circulatory system. This form of hypoxia occurs when the cells of your tissues are unable to take up or use the oxygen that has been delivered properly to them by your blood. This condition is not considered true hypoxia because the oxygenation levels of your tissues may be normal or even above normal. Reasons for histotoxic hypoxia include cyanide poisoning, use of certain narcotics, and alcohol consumption.

Cyanide leads to histotoxic hypoxia by blocking a necessary reaction for the cellular usage of oxygen. There may be more than enough oxygen available to the cells of your tissues, but once they have been poisoned by cyanide they simply cannot use it. The use of narcotics has long been known to have an inhibitory effect on oxygen uptake,[11] while the consumption of alcohol alters the permeability of cells in a way that also leads to histotoxic hypoxia.

INCREASING YOUR OXYGEN LEVELS

Over 1.5 million people die each year from heart conditions, and heart attacks result from the failure of the heart muscle to receive adequate supplies of oxygen.[12] It has been suggested that much of the time we do not have enough oxygen in our bodies to support the daily functions of all our internal and external organs optimally. Simply put, we need more oxygen. So, how do we get it?

You cannot survive for more than a few minutes without oxygen because your cells cannot store adequate amounts of oxygen for more than a few minutes. Therefore, you need to acquire oxygen from your environment constantly. Thankfully, there are a number of ways in which you may increase the oxygen levels in your blood and improve your health as a result. The following are simple, natural methods to help you boost your oxygen levels, help your circulation, and improve your body's ability to absorb and use oxygen more efficiently.

Get Some Exercise

It should come as no surprise that exercising regularly helps increase your oxygen levels. As you exercise, your breathing rate increases and deepens. The more you engage in exercise, the better your lungs will be able to absorb oxygen. Even light exercise can lead to improvements in lung capacity, but to be sure that your blood is getting saturated with oxygen optimally, you should try to work out moderately and regularly. Avoid sitting for long period s of time, and if you must sit for extended lengths of time, try to stand up every couple of hours and stretch your legs. Just standing up will provide you with benefits.

When you work out at a moderate pace, your body burns oxygen at a faster rate than it normally does. This cause carbon dioxide levels in your body to increase, which results in your brain sending signals to boost your respiration rate in order to acquire a greater supply of oxygen. Your lungs and heart then work to take in and transport more oxygen. Exercise can even benefit people with low oxygen levels due to pulmonary disease.

Do your best to increase you aerobic exercise, as this type of exercise is known to elevate your heart rate and breathing rate in a way that allows your body to sustain itself for an extended period of exertion, unlike anaerobic exercise, which causes you to become out of breath quickly. Good examples of aerobic exercise include walking, jogging, hiking, swimming, dancing, and bicycling.

In addition to increasing your oxygen levels, aerobic exercise helps your lymphatic system, which is responsible for removing waste and other toxins from your body, function properly. A sedentary lifestyle is detrimental to your lymphatic system, which does not have a pump to circulate lymph in the same manner that your heart pumps blood throughout your body. Your lymphatic system relies on gravity and movement to circulate lymph. Thus, exercise can improve your health not only by increasing your oxygen levels but also by helping your lymphatic system do its job.

If you are out of shape, start slowly and build up to a regimen of moderate exercise. Don't overdo it. Begin by getting ten to fifteen minutes of light aerobic exercise three to four times a week. Work your way up to getting at least thirty minutes of moderate aerobic exercise every day. It takes time to get in shape, so try not to be impatient. Set fitness goals for yourself and then gradually modify these goals to increase the effort required to reach them.

If you have a friend who could join you in your exercise routines, invite this person along. It helps to have support and encouragement. And if you live in a smoggy urban area and wish to job outside, try to find a park with lots of trees and plants in which to do so. The greenery will help to filter out some of the pollutants in the air and provide you with higher oxygen levels.

Get Some Fresh Air

When the air in your home is stagnant, it lacks an optimal amount of oxygen. While modern housing construction techniques have allowed builders to eliminate drafts, they have also made it more likely that a house will have stale air. In light of this fact, perhaps the easiest thing you can do to increase your oxygen levels is open your windows and let some fresh air into your home. If you have trees and foliage nearby, they will boost the amounts of oxygen in the air that blows in.

If you happen to live in a high-smog area, you could always look into getting an air-filtration system for your home. Gas fumes and other emissions contain chemicals that can interfere with your body's ability to absorb and transport oxygen. If you are able to avoid areas where these chemicals are prevalent in the air, such as roads with a lot of traffic congestion, then do so. If you live in an urban area, as so many of us do, this may be tough to accomplish. If this is the case for you, be sure to plant trees and shrubs where you can outside your home, and to get a few house plants. Plants, as you know, take in carbon dioxide and release oxygen, so having a few in your home should increase the amount of oxygen in your indoor air supply.

Drink More Water

The water molecule comprises oxygen, so if you increase your intake of water, you will boost the oxygen in your body. An added benefit of water consumption is that it facilitates the transportation of blood and other bodily fluids, helping in cellular respiration and the removal of toxins from your body.

If you would like to drink something else in addition to water, you could always make fresh vegetable and fruit smoothies or juice, thus receiving the benefits of the vitamins and minerals these foods contain. Try to avoid too many sweet juices, as they have very high sugar contents, which will increase acidity in the body and potentially reduce oxygen levels.

Eat Better

Eating more leafy greens and green vegetables, such as kale, spinach, broccoli, and celery, can raise the oxygen levels in your blood because these foods are rich in oxygen content. As well, plant foods are alkaline instead of acidic, and following a more alkaline diet may also help increase oxygen levels in your body. Reducing the number of processed foods and animal products you consume may also help in this endeavor.

Eating a healthy diet of plant foods also provides your body with high levels of antioxidants, such as vitamin A, vitamin C, and vitamin E. Antioxidants allow your body to manage oxygen more effectively so that it enters your bloodstream in optimal amounts. Choose blueberries, cranberries, strawberries, red kidney beans, walnuts, or pecans, which are all high in antioxidants, when you are making your meals or looking for a snack.

As you are aware, the hemoglobin in your red blood cells is responsible for binding oxygen and carrying it to your tissues. When you lack sufficient hemoglobin in your blood, as is the case in anemia, you will thus suffer from low oxygen levels in your body. Adequate amounts of iron are required for hemoglobin production, which is why iron deficiency is such a common cause of anemia. Thankfully, there are numerous iron-rich foods you can eat to ensure healthy hemoglobin levels.

Although animal meats are relatively high in iron, you don't have to eat hamburgers ate every meal to boost your iron count, nor should you, as animal products are acidic and can be detrimental to your health when consumed in high amounts. Leafy greens, broccoli, lentils, black beans, kidney beans, cashews, pistachios, and sunflower seeds can all improve iron deficiency and boost blood oxygen levels. Depending on your age and sex, you will need approximately 8 to 18 mg of iron in your diet each day to stave off anemia. There are about 2 mg in half a cup of cooked kidney beans or one ounce of cashews, while half a cup of cooked lentils contains a little over 3 mg. When consuming iron-rich foods, it is helpful to pair them with foods high in vitamin C, as this vitamin aids in iron absorption.

Essential fatty acids have been shown to increase the oxygen-carrying capacity of the hemoglobin in your blood, ease the flow of your blood, and boost your metabolism. As such, seeds and nuts, which contain essential fatty acids, should be added to your diet. Good choices include walnuts, pumpkin seeds, flax seeds, hemp seeds, and chia seeds.

Finally, reduce the amount of salt in your diet. A low-sodium diet can result in increased oxygen in your body.

Try Oxygen Therapy

When you injure your body, healing cannot occur without appropriate amounts of oxygen reaching these injured tissues. For those afflicted with conditions that negatively affect their circulatory systems, oxygen cannot adequately nourish damaged areas, so the natural healing abilities of their bodies cannot function properly.

Oxygen therapy is the dispensing of oxygen as part of medical care, and it can be used in a variety of scenarios, either chronic or acute. Oxygen first aid has been used as an emergency treatment for diving injuries for years. Nurses supply and administer oxygen to patients daily. In fact, oxygen is a serious drug if you are in the medical profession. Oxygen therapy may be utilized to:

- improve the speed of rehabilitation after serious illness.

- improve the speed of wound healing and contribute to the normalization of low blood pressure.

- significantly improve bronchial asthma and shortness of breath.

- significantly improve degenerative phenomena in eyes.

- significantly improve side effects of conventional cancer therapies.

- stabilize immune system for cancer prevention and against cancer relapse.

- improve circulatory disorders in extremities.

- improve general circulation stability.

- produce positive effects in the treatment of certain liver diseases.

- lower frequency and severity of migraine attacks.

- lower frequency of angina-pectoris attacks.

- lower side effects and increase main effects of medications.

- lower susceptibility to disease.

- improve oxygen reserve associated with lack of exercise after serious illnesses.

- strengthen respiratory muscles in pulmonary emphysema patients.

Depending on your medical condition, you may even require an oxygen machine in your home or a portable oxygen tank.

Breathe Better

When it comes to increasing your oxygen levels, breathing must sound like a no-brainer. But breathing properly is quite another matter, and one that must be addressed. In fact, it has been reported that improper breathing habits may lead to reductions in blood oxygen levels of as much as 20 percent.

One of the first things you can do to breathe properly is improve your posture. When you slouch you also make it more difficult for your body to take in an optimal supply of oxygen. Try to make a habit of sitting up straight and walking with your shoulders back so that you can inhale more oxygen and thus raise the level of oxygen in your blood. Another easy adjustment you can make is to stop wearing tight clothing, which restricts your ability to breathe properly. Opt for loose clothing so that you can breathe in and out fully and without effort.

UJJAYI BREATHING

Breathing exercises known as *pranayama* are an important aspect of practicing yoga. The ujjayi pranayama is a form of deep breathing in which you breathe slowly through your nose while contracting your throat slightly, using your diaphragm to fill your lungs completely with each breath. The increased oxygen intake is meant to invigorate and relax you.

The name of this breathing technique comes from the Sanskrit word "ujjayi," which means "to be victorious," why is why it is also known as "victorious breath." More commonly, this breathing method is called "ocean breath" due to the sound created as the air passes through your somewhat narrowed airway. By practicing this pranayama regularly, using your diaphragm to control the length of your breaths, you will strengthen your diaphragm and increase your lung capacity over time.

Although most pranayamas must be performed in a sitting position or lying down, ujjayi may be used in combination with any yoga pose. Some poses may actually complement this deep-breathing practice, such as backbends, which lengthen your spine while allowing your lungs to expand and contract fully with each breath, helping to eliminate carbon dioxide, lactic acid, lymphatic fluid, and other waste from your body.

When you take shallow breaths, the amount of oxygen in your bloodstream is lowered. Breathing at a quicker pace may seem like a good way to bring more oxygen into your body, but the truth is that breathing slowly and deeply is the way to raise your blood oxygen levels. Aim to take about twelve breaths each minute, using your diaphragm to inhale and exhale rather than your chest, and breathing through your nose instead of your mouth. This technique will allow you to take more oxygen into your lungs, as it uses your entire lung capacity. Deep breathing is also known to relax your nervous system and improve your digestion.

The more you practice deep breathing, the better your lungs will function. Over time, you will actually increase the capacity of your lungs, making the oxygenation of your blood and body even more effective. Just a few of the noted benefits of proper oxygenation are stress reduction, increased energy, elevated brain function, and a healthier life.

Laugh More

Laughter has many benefits, a major one of which is that it increases oxygen levels in your body by encouraging you to breathe in larger amounts of air than you might normally take in. In addition to boosting the amount of oxygen in your blood, laughter improves digestion and aids in the movement of lymph throughout your body, thus helping rid your body of waste and strengthening your immune system.

Get a Massage

Massages are not only relaxing but also increase circulation in your body, allowing the oxygen in your blood to reach the tissues that need it more easily. Understandably, massage also aids in the movement of lymph throughout your body, helping flush waste from your system.

Meditate, Pray

The practice of meditation, which typically involves taking deep breaths and focusing on your breathing, can be of great assistance in both oxygen intake and stress reduction. Daily prayer can also improve your oxygen intake while helping you find peace and serenity. Even simply sitting quietly and slowly breathing in and out can be immensely beneficial to your blood oxygen levels.

Avoid Cigarettes, Alcohol, and Drugs

If you are trying increase the amount of oxygen in your blood but you are a smoker, then quit now. Get help if you need it, but quit. Smoking decreases the level of oxygen in your blood. As long as you continue to smoke, other oxygen-boosting methods will not be as effective.

In addition, due to the mechanism by which they are metabolized and removed from your body, alcohol and drugs can negatively impact the amount of oxygen in your blood. For this reason and many others, use of alcohol and drugs should be avoided.

CONCLUSION

Blood transports oxygen, which is critically important to your health and wellness. A shortage of oxygen in the body, hypoxia, may occur for various reasons, some of which you can take steps to avoid. There are numerous ways to increase the amount of oxygen you inhale and absorb and therefore raise your blood oxygen levels. Easy steps you can take include open your windows, wearing loose clothing, improving your posture and learning how to breathe properly. Eating better and getting more exercise may be slightly harder methods of elevating your blood oxygen levels, but once you notice how good you feel after making these adjustments, you'll wish you had done so sooner. Finally, oxygen therapy can be used in both chronic and acute medical care, which just goes to show you how powerful a substance it is. Any changes you can make that lead to better breathing and increased oxygen capacity in your lungs will also lead to greater overall health.

PART THREE

Detoxifying Your Blood

Part Three of this book is a comprehensive guide to taking your well-being into your own hands and supporting the cleansing of your blood through diet and fasting, dietary supplementation, and complementary therapies. Chapter 7 details the ways in which dietary choices can encourage healthy blood and overall wellness or keep you from attaining good health. Chapter 8 provides specific advice on supplements that may positively affect the different aspects of your body's detoxification system, which include your organs of detoxification (skin, kidneys, liver, and intestines). Chapter 9 wraps everything up by reviewing complementary therapies that may be used to promote the detoxification process, including sauna therapy, hydrotherapy, massage therapy, chelation therapy, and meditation.

7

Foods and Fasts for Blood Cleansing

Just as poor dietary practices—such as eating too much salt, sugar, or saturated fat, or consuming too many calories—can lead to various chronic diseases, including type 2 diabetes and cardiovascular disease, what you eat can affect your body's defenses against exposure to harmful substances. The foods you eat can help cleanse your blood and promote your overall well-being, or they can add to the burden that an unhealthy diet places on your body.[1] We all know that dietary habits such as eating vegetables and drinking plenty of water can keep us healthy, but most of us don't really understand why this is the case. This chapter details the ways in which dietary choices can help you maintain healthy blood and thus a healthy body, and the ways in which they can hold you back from living in a state of wellness.

FOODS AND DIETARY PRACTICES THAT PROMOTE TOXIC BUILDUP

In terms of avoiding foods and dietary practices that can lead to a buildup of toxins in your body, there are some obvious choices you can make. First, take it easy on the junk food. Second, choose organic foods over conventional foods as often as possible, since conventional foods are more likely to contain pesticides and other harmful compounds. (See "Organic Foods" on page 137.) Third, include plenty of fiber in your diet, as a low-fiber diet can lead to constipation. At best, constipation is inconvenient and unpleasant. At worst, long-term constipation can contribute towards inefficient detoxification and the development of serious medical conditions.

Constipation

According to the National Institute of Diabetes and Digestive and Kidney Diseases (NIDDK), constipation is defined as having a bowel movement fewer than three times per week, although others contend that experiencing fewer than a daily bowel movement is indicative of constipation, and still others say that experiencing fewer than two or three bowel movements daily should be considered constipation.[2] In any case, authorities agree that the stools of constipated individuals are usually hard, dry, small in size, and difficult to eliminate. Some people who are constipated find it painful to have a bowel movement and often experience straining, bloating, and the sensation of a full bowel. Essentially, people are considered to be constipated if they experience two or more of the following symptoms:[3]

- Straining during a bowel movement more than 25 percent of the time.

- Hard stools more than 25 percent of the time.

- Incomplete evacuation more than 25 percent of the time.

Unfortunately, constipation is commonplace. In the United States more than 4 million people experience frequent constipation, accounting for 2.5 million physician visits a year.

Stool will move through your colon too slowly if peristalsis—which refers to the involuntary movements of intestinal muscles that shift the contents of the intestines along—is sluggish, resulting in constipation. Most commonly, this sluggishness is caused by a lack of adequate fiber in your diet. Americans eat an average of 5 to 14 grams of fiber daily.[4] This falls significantly short of the Food and Nutrition Board of the Institute of Medicine's adequate intake recommendations for fiber of 38 grams daily for men fifty years of age or older and 25 grams daily for women fifty years of age or younger, and 30 grams daily for men over fifty and 21 grams daily for women over fifty.[5]

The NIDDK has identified the following as common causes of constipation:[6]

- Abuse of laxatives

- Certain diseases or conditions, including stroke (most common)

- Changes in life or routine such as pregnancy, aging, or travel

- Chronic problems with intestinal function

- Dehydration

- Ignoring the urge to have a bowel movement

- Irritable bowel syndrome

- Lack of physical activity (especially in the elderly)

- Medications

- Milk

- Problems with the colon and rectum

Some well-known health ramifications of constipation include hemorrhoids, which may result from straining to have a bowel movement, and anal fissures—tears in the skin around the anus—which may occur when hard stool stretches the sphincter muscle. Anal fissures may cause rectal bleeding, which may appear as bright red streaks on the surface of stool. Sometimes straining causes rectal prolapse, which refers protrusion of the rectum from the anus. This condition may lead to secretion of mucus from the anus. Constipation may also cause fecal impaction, in which hard stool is packed in the intestine so tightly that the normal pushing action of the colon is not enough to expel the stool. Fecal impaction occurs most often in children and older adults.[7]

In addition, there are other, more serious, conditions that may occur as a result of constipation, including increased permeability of your gut, which raises your risk of certain molecules entering your bloodstream that should not be there. Gut permeability, or intestinal permeability, describes how easily the lining of your gut allows material to pass through it and into your capillaries, where it enters your bloodstream, travels throughout your body, and may lead to health issues. A gut whose lining has been compromised and allows undesirable material to pass through it into the bloodstream is also known as a *leaky gut,* and those who suffer from this problem are considered to have *leaky gut syndrome.*

When substances such as certain protein molecules and polypeptide molecules penetrate the normal mucosal barrier that lines your intestinal tract and begin to build up in your circulatory system, your immune system may start to recognize them, setting off inflammatory reactions.[8] There are, in fact, a number of molecules that may lead to toxic, hormonal, or immunological reactions once they have accumulated in sufficient amounts in your bloodstream due to intestinal permeability.[9] Furthermore, gut permeability also has a relationship to constipation.

In a clinical study of fifty-seven patients with chronic constipation, this condition was found to be associated with striking changes in intestinal permeability and systemic immune response.[10] Therapy with a laxative was found to be associated with a return to immune system function within normal parameters, which led the study's authors to conclude that the undesirable changes in intestinal permeability and immune response had been caused by constipation.

Constipation can also have a profound effect on your intestinal flora. Intestinal flora, or gut flora, refers to the bacteria that live in your digestive tract. Gut flora can produce a number of compounds—some beneficial, such as immune system-stimulating substances;[11] and others harmful, such as carcinogens and tumor-promoting substances.[12] The type and quantity of these compounds are determined by the type and quantity of your gut flora.

If you evacuate your bowels infrequently, as is the case when you are constipated, undesirable gut flora is given a greater opportunity to wreak havoc. Internationally noted medical herbalist Simon Mills wrote, "A transit time double that of the primitive bowel means that there is approximately twice as much opportunity for toxic fermentation and for reabsorption."[13] In other words, our modern diet has extended the time it takes the human body to expel waste, which gives harmful compounds a chance to multiply and thrive, damaging your immune system function and possibly allowing dangerous substances to enter your bloodstream.

Harmful Interactions

Aside from the dangers of constipation, it is also important to consider the interactions different compounds may have with each other in your bloodstream, some of which may negatively affect your health and should be avoided, if possible. Just as certain drugs interact negatively with other drugs in your bloodstream, certain foods have problematic effects on pharmaceuticals in your bloodstream as well.[14]

One of the best-known drug-nutrient interactions is that between grapefruit juice (and other citrus juices) and pharmaceuticals, which any pharmacist can tell you about.[15] It is widely known that grapefruit juice inhibits the action of cytochrome P450 enzymes and affects particular phase III proteins. In doing so, grapefruit juice significantly hinders your body's ability to absorb and metabolize drugs, causing them to build up in your bloodstream to possibly disastrous results. Consequently, taking daily medicine with a glass of grapefruit or other citrus juice is highly discouraged.

FOODS AND DIETARY PRACTICES THAT PROMOTE DETOXIFICATION

Foods help promote blood cleansing by providing sources of vital natural compounds that help the body rid itself of unwelcome foreign compounds and unwanted byproducts of normal physiological processes. According to the Academy of Nutrition and Dietetics, there are a handful of dietary choices you can make to ensure these harmful substances do not build up in your system.[16]

Relieving Constipation

You may prevent or alleviate constipation by increasing your intake of dietary fiber, which softens and add bulk to your stool, easing its passage through your colon.[17] Sources of fiber that have been most consistently found to increase stool bulk and shorten transit time include wheat bran, fruit, and vegetables.[18] Sufficient fluid intake is also required to maximize the stool-softening effect of increased fiber intake.[19] In addition to increasing fiber intake, drinking at least sixty-four ounces of fluid daily is usually recommended to help prevent or treat constipation.[20]

Most people who are mildly constipated do not need laxatives. For those who have made diet and lifestyle changes and are still constipated, however, laxatives may be recommended by a doctor to retrain chronically sluggish bowels.

Exercise also helps relieve constipation by accelerating your breathing and heart rate. Increases in your breathing and heart rate stimulate peristalsis, thus helping your body expel fecal matter more quickly.[21] In addition, by decreasing the time it takes food to move through your large intestine, exercise also limits the amount of water absorbed from your stool by your body, thus preventing the occurrence of hard, dry stools, which are harder to pass. Physical activity has even been shown to increase the frequency of bowel movements in constipated older adults.[22]

Supporting Detoxification Mechanisms

Drinking enough water to maintain adequate hydration not only helps relieve constipation but also supports your body's other detoxification mechanisms, as does eating five to nine servings of fruit and vegetables every day. You should also consume an adequate amount of protein, which is critical to maintaining optimum levels of a substance known as glutathione. Glutathione-related enzymes are crucial to the detoxification process. To determine an adequate amount of daily protein (in grams) for yourself, multiply your weight in pounds by 0.36. This will provide you with your recommended protein intake per day.[23]

Certain foods are known to support the detoxification pathways of your body and so should be added to your diet, including cruciferous vegetables (cabbage, cauliflower, broccoli, etc.), berries, artichokes, garlic, onions, leeks, turmeric, and milk thistle. Green tea also supports your body's detoxification mechanisms. Fermented foods such as kefir, yogurt, kimchi, and sauerkraut encourage a good probiotic environment in your gut, which also helps your body manage harmful substances. Finally, you should consider taking a multivitamin if you feel there are gaps in your diet, as a number of vitamins and minerals are vital to the proper functioning of your body's detoxification processes.

A diet that is high in vegetable content is recommended because it provides compounds that aid your liver in detoxifying your body. In particular, a high-vegetable diet increases your levels of cytochrome P450 enzymes, which play a role in detoxification phases I and III.[24] (See page 53.) In addition, vegetables contain a considerable amount of soluble fiber, which is essential to maintaining healthy gut bacteria and thus a healthy immune system. Fiber has also been shown to repair gut permeability and could help prevent *bacteremia*, which refers to the presence of bacteria in your blood.[25] Although vegetables of all kinds are good for you, cruciferous vegetables seem to offer the widest range of therapeutic benefits.[26]

Cruciferous vegetables have been shown to boost detoxification and contain anticancer compounds, including sulforaphane and indole-3-carbinol.[27,28] In fact, research has shown that indole-3-carbinol promotes healthy cell division and cell replication, helping to prevent breast, cervical, endometrial, colorectal, and prostate cancers, while also supporting your body's detoxification process. And indole-3-carbinol is only one of several compounds found in vegetables that might play a valuable role in healthy cell division.[29]

Indole-3-carbinol also helps support your liver's ability to metabolize estrogen and dispose of toxins. Your liver converts estradiol, the major form of estrogen, into one of two metabolites. One of these metabolites is good, and one is bad. The bad metabolite can interfere with healthy cell division in the breast and cervix, potentially leading to cancer, while the good metabolite does not have this effect. Indole-3-carbinol encourages your liver to convert estradiol into the good metabolite. In this way, indole-3-carbinol may support healthy cell division and help you avoid cancer.[30] In addition, research indicates that indole-3-carbinol has antioxidant properties, which may also protect you against cancer.[31]

Other important food components that promote detoxification include the amino acids methionine and cysteine. These amino acids are needed to create metallothionein, a family of proteins that are responsible for binding and clearing metallic elements such as cadmium, mercury, silver, and arsenic from your bloodstream. As well, insufficient dietary methionine leads to a loss of S-adenosyl methionine, on which certain methylation reactions that boost glutathione levels and help detoxification are dependent.

In addition, cysteine is a building block for glutathione, which, as mentioned earlier, is crucial to keeping your blood healthy. Without glutathione, your body's ability to eliminate various toxins and prevent cellular damage caused by free radicals would be severely compromised.[32] These amino acids may be found in virtually any protein-rich food; plant sources such as garlic, red peppers, onions, oats, and sprouted lentils; as well as whey and rice protein powders.

The medical establishment's understanding of how particular dietary components help cleanse your blood has developed over at least three decades. It started with research published in the late 70s that showed dietary intake of cruciferous vegetables altered the metabolism of drugs in the body, increasing the rate at which the body clears drugs from its system.[33] As research continued and knowledge increased, it was discovered that certain dietary components induce a number of phase II detoxification actions.[34] Some researchers even used the phase II detoxification enzyme *quinone reductase* as a marker for detoxification activity, as many other phase II enzymes were shown to be active in association with quinone reductase.[35]

Another important step forward was the recognition that quinone reductase and many other phase II enzymes all contain a particular DNA sequence that plays a role in phase II detoxification: the antioxidant response element, or ARE.[36] Apparently, certain antioxidants and other compounds are able to activate genes that contain the ARE.[37] Although the ARE is far from being the only DNA sequence that helps regulate phase II detoxification, it appears to be the one most frequently affected by diet. Examples of dietary compounds that promote the production of quinone reductase include sulforaphane from broccoli and curcumin from the curry ingredient turmeric.[38]

Ongoing research continues to explain the ways in which phase II detoxification enzymes and phase III detoxification systems are activated by so many food components.[39] As it turns out, there are ARE sequences present on a number of genes involved in phase III as well.[40] For some reason, however, the ARE does not appear to be present on phase I genes. Nevertheless, other dietary components activate phase I enzymes through a separate DNA sequence referred to as the xenobiotic response element, or XRE. Many phase II enzymes also contain this sequence, which explains the coordinated activity of phase I enzymes with a number of phase II enzymes in response to dietary elements that trigger the XRE.[41]

One such element is indole-3-carbinol, which was discussed

earlier. Indole-3-carbinol can generate compounds in the acid environment of the stomach that activate the XRE sequence, including 3,3'-diindolylmethane, often referred to as DIM.[42] This action triggers activity of phase I and phase II detoxification enzymes. In some genes, the ARE and XRE sequences are in such close proximity that if separate food components activate both at the same time, they can interact cooperatively, maintaining prolonged activity and detoxification.[43]

Now that we've reviewed the mechanisms by which food components act, it is easier to understand how various food components boost the effectiveness of your body's detoxification systems. It also makes sense that whole foods and mixtures may provide greater effects than single components.[44] In addition to certain vegetables such as cruciferous vegetables, onions, red peppers, oats, and sprouted lentils; spices such as turmeric (or curry, which contains turmeric); and the protein obtained from meat or protein powders; green tea also supports detoxification enzymes.[45]

CHOOSING A DIET

The main thing to remember when using your diet to promote detoxification is to eat plenty of produce (fruit and vegetables). In other words, the inclusion of lots of fruit and vegetables in every meal should be inherent to whichever diet you follow. As well, eating a large amount of saturated fat is not conducive to keeping your blood healthy. So, when it comes to maintaining the effectiveness of your body's natural detoxification systems, which diet plans should you try and which should you avoid?

■ MEDITERRANEAN DIET

The Mediterranean diet includes large amounts of fruit, vegetables, bread and other whole grain cereals, potatoes, beans, nuts, and seeds. As such, it should supply sufficient levels of the previously mentioned compounds that support your detoxification

ORGANIC FOODS

It is important to choose organic foods as often as possible, as they seem to have higher nutritional value in addition to their lower pesticide content.[46,47] Most people, doctors, and government regulatory agencies do not take the health impact of the pesticide residues found on food supplies seriously enough. The estrogenic effects of pesticides may accelerate breast cancer and other hormone-sensitive cancers, and this reaction is magnified when more than one type of pesticide is present or when pesticide ingestion is combined with the consumption of large quantities of alcohol. An Israeli study, in fact, associated a drop in the incidence of breast cancer among Israeli women with a new law prohibiting the use of pesticides.[48]

pathways. It should also contain a beneficial amount of fiber, which, as you know, is vital to your gut health as well as your overall well-being. Furthermore, dairy products, fish, poultry, and wine are consumed in low to moderate amounts and little red meat is eaten in the Mediterranean diet. These characteristics keep it in line with the recommendations outlined in this chapter on how to maintain healthy blood.

Research has shown that the Mediterranean diet reduces mortality rates and rates of fatal and nonfatal heart attack,[49] provides protection against coronary heart disease,[50] and helps control blood glucose levels.[51] The Mediterranean diet is generally a good choice.

■ SOUTH BEACH DIET

The South Beach Diet was designed prevent heart disease but gained in popularity as a means to lose weight.[52] A primary principle of the South Beach Diet is to replace "bad carbohydrates" with "good carbohydrates," and "bad fats" with "good fats." Consequently, the South Beach Diet favors relatively unprocessed foods such as vegetables, beans, and whole grains. This diet plan also avoids trans fats and discourages consumption of saturated fats, replacing them with foods rich in omega-3 fatty acids and other unsaturated fats. Overall, the South Beach diet seems to be a good option for supporting detoxification. It has also been shown to promote heart health and a healthy weight.[53]

■ ATKINS DIET

Created by Dr. Robert Atkins, the Atkins diet is a low-carbohydrate plan that is relatively high in fat and protein. Part of the rationale for lowering consumption of carbohydrates is to prevent an excess of glucose or other sugars being added to your body's metabolic system. In essence, Dr. Atkins proposed that the body regularly produces insulin to convert excess carbohydrates into body fat, and so that excess carbohydrates must be eliminated so as not to create more fat.[54] While a number of scientific studies on this low-carbohydrate diet lend support to the claim that this approach can lead to weight loss, the high content of saturated fat in this diet make it a bad idea for supporting healthy blood.[55,56]

■ PALEO DIET

The Paleo diet, or Paleolithic diet, is a fad diet based on eating foods similar to those that might have been consumed during the Paleolithic era, which dates from approximately 2.5 million to 10,000 years ago. Typically, this includes lean meats, fish, fruits, vegetables, nuts, and seeds, which are foods that could have been obtained by hunting and gathering. In addition, the Paleo diet limits foods that became common when farming emerged about 10,000 years ago, such as dairy products, legumes, and grains.[57] Although the digestive abilities of modern humans are different from those of Paleolithic humans (thereby undermining the premise that we should be eating like our ancestors in order to obtain good health), the Paleo diet may still be acceptable for supporting detoxification, as long as the meats consumed are, in fact, lean.

■ PLANT-BASED DIETS

Simply put, a vegan diet consists of all plant-based foods. It does not include any animal-based foods—this means no meat, fish, poultry, eggs, or dairy. Also a plant-based diet, vegetarianism may or may not include eggs or dairy, but does not include meat. People who consume dairy and eggs as their exclusive sources of animal protein are known as lacto-ovo vegetarians. As well, pescetarians, whose diet includes fish and seafood but no other animal flesh (although they may still eat eggs and dairy), may also consider themselves vegetarians of a sort.

Both vegan and vegetarian diets offer several benefits, such as a reduction in risk of cardiovascular disease. Plant-based diets are also associated with lower body mass index (BMI); lower plasma concentrations of lipids, lipoproteins, glucose, insulin, and C-reactive protein; and lower blood pressure (both systolic and diastolic) and thickness of the internal diameter of the carotid artery (a measure of heart disease risk) than are other ways of eating.[58]

Long-term benefits of this type of diet were also seen in a seventeen-year observational study of vegetarians and other health conscious people. Results demonstrated that daily consumption of fresh fruit was associated with significantly reduced mortality from ischaemic heart disease and cerebrovascular disease.[59] Overall the individuals in the study had a mortality about half that of the general population. Nevertheless, it is important that vegetarians consume adequate amounts of protein—even if they are acquired from plant sources, such as beans—to support detoxification.

■ CALORIC RESTRICTION AND FASTING

Caloric restriction—that is, eating fewer calories—has been found to be of benefit in maintaining tissue glutathione levels during aging compared to the typical excess of calories consumed in the typical American diet. In addition, caloric restriction supports a more rapid rebound of glutathione synthesis following loss of glutathione after *ischemia,* which refers to an inadequate blood supply to an organ or part of the body, especially the heart muscles.[60] Since low glutathione levels reduce your ability to control oxidative damage and are a key concern as you age, the benefits of caloric restriction should be seriously considered as you grow older.

In addition, the effects of calorie restriction (eating between 70 and 80 percent of your typical intake) on health and longevity have been extensively studied and have demonstrated that eating less may boost your immune system and have a major impact on reducing your risk of chronic disease.[61] Caloric restriction may also lead to improvements in clearance of unwanted byproducts by your liver and your body's overall capacity for detoxification. Of course, acute caloric restriction, or fasting (i.e., starvation), has very different effects than does limiting caloric intake over a period of time. Complete removal of food will rapidly result in insufficient dietary methionine in addition to many other physiological difficulties.[62]

Fasting on water for a very short period of time, however, can provide important benefits. Without food to process, the metabolic machinery of your body is able to focus on cleansing your blood and lymph.[63] Although water fasting may not be a suitable choice for someone whose health is severely compromised, research has shown caloric restriction and fasting may alleviate hypertension,[64] diabetes,[65] epilepsy,[66] and rheumatoid arthritis.[67] Research has shown, in fact, that caloric restriction may be the most powerful way known yet to extend lifespan.[68,69] While high glucose and insulin levels damage mitochondria—the "powerhouses of the cell," as they are otherwise known—studies have shown that limiting caloric intake reduces oxidative stress within these structures.[70,71] In addition, a few animal studies have indicated that caloric restriction may help reduce risks of age-related diseases associated with impaired fat metabolism.[72]

Short-term fasting appears to have measurable benefits for your immune system,[73] allowing your intestines and liver, which are key sites of immune function, to rest. Research indicates that fasting for thirty-six to sixty hours can significantly increase the power of white blood cells to destroy pathogenic bacteria,[74] which may help restore impaired immune response.[75] Studies have also shown that caloric restriction can reduce cellular damage by inhibiting the formation of reactive oxygen species by certain white blood cells.[76,77]

In terms of long-term fasting, caution is advised, as it can deprive your body of nutrients that are critical to your health. While a two-day water fast is safe for most people, there are those with certain medical conditions who should avoid fasting altogether, including diabetics, hypoglycemics, and severely nutritionally deficient individuals. The most common risks associated with fasting are low blood sugar and low blood pressure with vertigo (dizziness), sometimes resulting in fainting. While these reactions are generally harmless, they are not pleasant, and may result in harm from a fall. Should you decide to fast, take extra care when standing up from a sitting position or getting out of a bed or bathtub. If faintness or vertigo does not go away within a few minutes, speak to your health practitioner.[78]

It should be noted that there is a big difference between following a two-day fast and fasting for a prolonged period of time. Research suggests that fasting for an extended amount of time can reduce your body's stores of glutathione, making it more susceptible to aging and disease. Long-term fasting can also hinder phase I of your body's detoxification process.[79] As a general rule, therefore, if you are fasting, try to avoid exposure to harmful chemicals as much as possible, since a lack of dietary protein will make your liver unable to process toxins optimally due to a resultant insufficiency of methionine and cysteine, which are vital to your body's detoxification pathways.

After a two-day water fast, when reintroducing food into your life, do so with a simple diet of rice, fruit, and vegetables for the first five days. This simple diet, similar to the type used to address allergic, behavioral, or digestive problems,[80] provides enough calories to sustain a person but is very easy on the intestinal environment to allow optimal rest. There are two reasons to follow a vegetarian diet for these first five days. First, a vegetarian diet contains fewer potential food allergens that may cause reactions in your intestinal tissues. Second, increased vegetable intake provides more soluble fiber, which prevents constipation; bioflavonoids and other antioxidants, which support a healthy immune system; and complex carbohydrates, which provide sustained energy. Some people may experience fatigue while on the on this five-day regimen, but this symptom may be corrected by adding rice- or whey-based protein shakes to your diet. If this addition doesn't do the trick, take heart in the fact that your fatigue should dissipate upon once you resume eating protein-rich foods.[81]

CONCLUSION

The Academy of Nutrition and Dietetics recommendations on how to support your body's natural detoxification mechanisms make good sense. Caloric restriction and an occasional two-day fast can also help support blood cleansing, and certain diets are more advantageous than others in terms of filling your plate with the greatest number of foods that are beneficial to a healthy bloodstream. If you still have nutritional gaps in your diet after adjusting your meal plan to include better food choices, dietary supplements may be of use in your efforts to support your body's ability to detoxify itself.

8

Dietary Supplements That Support Detoxification

The right dietary supplements can have powerful, beneficial effects on your body's methods of detoxification. This chapter provides specific guidance regarding which compounds can make a major impact on different aspects of these processes, and thus a major impact on your blood as well.

By now, no doubt, you are familiar with your major organs of detoxification: skin, kidneys, liver, and intestines. The roles of your skin and kidneys are relatively simple in comparison to the cleansing mechanisms associated with your liver and intestines. Your skin excretes certain toxins through sweat to a limited extent, including heavy metals and chemicals such as BPA. Your kidneys utilize your urine to rid itself of a broad array of other unwanted substances. Even so, a large number of toxins in your system are fat-soluble compounds, which means they must first be made water-soluble by your liver before they can be excreted through your urine. Therefore, the lion's share of your body's overall detoxification process takes place in your liver and, to a lesser extent, in your intestines.

Nevertheless, finding ways to support each aspect of your body's natural cleansing ability is always a good idea, and there are dietary supplements that can help your skin, kidneys, liver, and intestines function optimally.

■ SUPPORTING SKIN DETOXIFICATION

Skin is the largest organ of the human body as well as the boundary between your vital organs and the environment. As such, skin is not only subject to the internal aging process but must also deal with various external stressors. This combination leads to distinct structural changes to this organ, affecting not only its youthful appearance but also its various physiological functions. As skin ages, skin permeability decreases, normal lipid and sweat production slows, and immune function processes are delayed.[1]

As it turns out, the primary causes of skin aging are losses of collagen and elastin proteins (the fundamental components of connective tissue in your skin) and glycation of collagen and elastin.[2] Glycation refers to the bonding of a sugar molecule, such as glucose or fructose, to a lipid molecule or a protein molecule. When glycation occurs in association with collagen or elastin, protein molecules, the results, understandably, are a loss of skin elasticity and the formation of wrinkles.[3] Glycation can also have adverse effects on skin permeability and sweat production. Considering the fact that glycation of collagen and elastin may start in a person as young as twenty years old, and that collagen and elastin levels in skin decrease with age, it is advisable to address this issue with the correct supplements. In this case, the correct supplements include glucosamine hydrochloride, cherry blossom extract, and lemon balm extract.[4]

Glucosamine Hydrochloride

Although this supplement is used primarily to treat arthritis, in animal research and laboratory research on human cells, glucosamine has also been shown to help decrease the results of glycation.[5] Furthermore, glucosamine has been clinically shown to promote the production of collagen and have a positive effect on skin markers (both in the epidermal layer and the much thicker dermal layer beneath it) associated with age.[6] In addition, human clinical research has also demonstrated that glucosamine can increase the moisture content of skin, improve dry skin, decrease the scaliness of skin, and improve the smoothness of skin.[7] You may achieve these benefits by taking 1,500 mg of glucosamine hydrochloride daily.

Cherry Blossom Extract

Known as sakura flowers in Japan, cherry blossoms are a highly revered symbol of spring and renewal. This symbolism is apropos in connection with its botanical extract as well, which contains potent bioactive compounds that produce beneficial anti-glycation effects on skin.[8] In fact, human clinical research has shown that cherry blossom extract can reduce skin AGEs, suppress loss of skin elasticity, reduce pigmentation and reddish areas, suppress enlargement of pore area, reduce dryness of skin, and improve skin smoothness.[9] The clinically effective dose is 150 mg per day.

Lemon Balm

Although generally used for its calming effects, lemon balm is an herb that may actually play a particularly valuable role where collagen glycation is concerned. To understand why this may be the case, it should be noted that glycation causes cross-linking of collagen proteins in the skin. This cross-linking makes it extremely difficult to replace damaged collagen in skin. Thankfully, lemon balm contains a natural compound called rosmarinic acid, which, in laboratory research, has demonstrated an ability to break the bonds between cross-linked proteins caused by glycation.[10]

Additional research has shown that lemon balm may help reduce protein glycation and counter changes in collagen caused by glycation.[11] Unsurprisingly, human research has demonstrated that lemon balm can improve skin elasticity, while other laboratory research has shown that lemon balm helps protect against skin damage caused by sun exposure.[12] In order for you to get an amount of rosmarinic acid sufficient to produce these benefits, a daily dosage of 1,240 mg of lemon balm (standardized for 5-percent rosmarinic acid) should be used.

■ SUPPORTING KIDNEY DETOXIFICATION

Generally, not much needs to be done to support kidney detoxification. The best approach is to drink a sufficient amount of water and other fluids daily. But how much is sufficient? According to the National Academies of Sciences, Engineering, and Medicine, an adequate daily water consumption goal is approximately 125 fluid ounces (3.7 liters) for the average adult male and approximately 91 fluid ounces (2.7 liters) for the average adult female. Don't panic, however, if these numbers seem daunting. Fluid intake requirements vary by individual and are dependent on numerous factors, including activity levels, geographic location, and temperature. As well, keep in mind that these recommendations factor in water derived from the food you consume, which typically accounts for 20 percent of your daily fluid intake. In truth, most people can achieve adequate hydration by simply drinking when they are thirsty.

■ SUPPORTING LIVER DETOXIFICATION

As discussed in Chapter 3, detoxification via your liver occurs in phases. After phase I reactions prepare toxins for the second part of the detoxification process, phase II takes over, and these molecules are conjugated with, or attached to, compounds such as glucuronic acid, sulfate, or glutathione, depending upon which of the six pathways of phase II is being utilized. Phase II renders these unwanted substances water soluble, allowing them to be excreted in urine or bile. The six pathways of phase II, as discussed in the following, include sulfation, glucuronidation, glutathione conjugation, acetylation, amino acid conjugation, and methylation.[13] You may support the function of each of these pathways by including certain dietary supplements in your daily routine.

Supporting the Sulfation Pathway

The conjugation of substances that contain sulfur-containing compounds takes place in the sulfation pathway. This pathway helps your body detoxify certain drugs and food additives and eliminate toxins from intestinal bacteria, steroid hormones, thyroid hormones, and neurotransmitters. As the sulfation pathway is the primary route for the elimination of neurotransmitters, which make possible the transmission of information between neurons, disruptions to this mechanism may contribute to the development of nervous system disorders.

N-Acetylcysteine

N-acetylcysteine (NAC) is a derivative of L-cysteine, a sulfur-containing amino acid. Research has shown that NAC can effectively support liver detox mechanisms, having molecules that contain sulfur, which is necessary for sulfation.[14] Since NAC is a precursor to glutathione, it can affect the glutathione pathway as well as the sulfation pathway. Research has also demonstrated that NAC promotes the excretion of heavy metals such as gold, silver, copper, mercury, lead, and arsenic. It is also used to treat poisoning by various substances, including carbon tetrachloride, acrylonitriles, halothane, paraquat, acetaldehyde, coumarin, and interferon.[15]

In its own right, NAC is an effective antioxidant, powerfully scavenging free radicals in your bloodstream. In addition to being extremely damaging to your cells, free radicals reduce intracellular and extracellular concentrations of glutathione. NAC supplementation is an efficient way to replenish glutathione and reduce damage caused by free radicals. In addition, human clinical research has demonstrated that NAC bolsters immunity when used for six months.[16]

NAC also has mucolytic properties. In other words, it makes mucus less thick and sticky, and thus easier to cough up. It supports effective expectoration (i.e., ejecting phlegm or mucus from the throat or lungs by coughing, hawking, or spitting) and reduces its frequency.[17] A daily NAC supplement of 600 mg should be sufficient to produce these benefits.

Berberine

Berberine is an alkaloid and a primary constituent of several plants, including European barberry, goldenseal, goldthread, Oregon grape, cork-tree, and tree turmeric. It has a long history of use in both Ayurvedic and Chinese medical traditions, and is well documented for its antimicrobial activity and its uses in managing blood glucose and lipid levels.

Berberine stimulates bile acid synthesis and bile secretion, which helps move the toxins processed in phase II into your intestines via your bile duct. Animal research has shown that berberine is able to promote the excretion of bilirubin with bile via the bile duct, and that it does so via the sulfation pathway.[18]

Human clinical research has shown that berberine is effective in significantly reducing fasting blood glucose and postprandial (after a meal) blood glucose levels, hemoglobin A1c (a measure of long-term glucose control), plasma triglycerides, total cholesterol, and LDL cholesterol in people with type 2 diabetes.[19] Other research has shown similar results, as well as the fact that berberine can reduce systolic and diastolic blood pressure. In patients with high cholesterol levels, berberine has shown the ability to reduce serum levels of cholesterol, triglycerides, and LDL cholesterol.[20] A sufficient daily intake of berberine is 1,000 to 1,500 mg split into two or three doses.

Caffeine

Sulfotransferases (SULTs) are sulfur-related enzymes that play an important role in the sulfation pathway. Caffeine, one of the most widely consumed chemicals in the world, is able to induce SULTs. In one study, caffeine was shown to induce SULTs in the livers and intestines of rats that had been given certain dosages of caffeine.[21] The researchers of this study concluded that "consumption of caffeine can induce drug metabolizing SULTs in drug detoxification tissues." Since most people consume caffeine in the form of coffee or tea, it is not strictly necessary to supplement with caffeine or caffeine-containing herbs. If additional support for the sulfation pathway is desired, however, 100 to150 mg of caffeine daily may be used.

Retinoic Acid (Vitamin A)

Research with rats has shown that *retinoic acid,* the bioactive form of vitamin A, is also able to induce SULTs. Likewise, research in human intestinal cancer cells has demonstrated a similar effect. It appears that retinoic acid actually activates genes to produce the SULTs.[22] Since retinoic acid is not readily available as a dietary supplement, the use of standard vitamin A is a viable substitute, since your body will convert vitamin A into retinoic acid. In addition, your body can convert beta-carotene into vitamin A, which can then be converted into retinoic acid—so beta-carotene may also be used for this purpose. A daily intake of 5,000 IU (1,500 mcg) is sufficient to support detoxification.

Supporting the Glucuronidation Pathway

Along the *glucuronidation pathway,* glucuronic acid is attached to particular toxins, including many commonly prescribed drugs, aspirin, menthol, synthetic vanilla, and food additives such as benzoates, as well as hormones such as estrogen, which are then excreted into your intestinal tract via bile to be eventually removed from your body. Beta-glucuronidase, a bacterial enzyme found in your intestines, can pose a challenge to this process, as it can break the bond that links glucuronic acid to a toxin. Once this bond has been broken, the toxin may be reabsorbed back into your bloodstream, thereby increasing the total number of toxins being handled by your liver and overburdening this organ of detoxification. There is, however, a way to inhibit beta-glucuronidase from breaking these important bonds, and it involves calcium d-glucarate.

Calcium D-Glucarate

D-glucaric acid is a natural substance found in many fruits and vegetables, including apples, grapefruit, broccoli, and Brussels sprouts. The calcium salt of D-glucaric acid, known as calcium D-glucarate, is available as a dietary supplement. Calcium D-glucarate has been shown to inhibit beta-glucuronidase.[23] In fact, according to data released from the University of Texas MD Anderson Cancer Center, calcium D-glucarate can inhibit beta-glucuronidase by 57 percent in your blood, 44 percent in your liver, 39 percent in your intestines, and 37 percent in your lungs.[24] Such an inhibition of beta-glucuronidase may do much to protect the action of the glucuronidation pathway. As a supplement, calcium-D-glucarate should be taken three times daily for a total intake of approximately 1,500 mg.[25]

Supporting the Glutathione Conjugation Pathway

Glutathione is a tripeptide composed of the amino acids cysteine, glutamic acid, and glycine. The glutathione conjugation pathway is vital to detoxifying and eliminating foreign compounds such as acetaminophen and nicotine, as well as heavy metals such as mercury, lead, and arsenic. The functioning of this pathway is dependent upon sufficient levels of glutathione.

Milk Thistle

In herbal medicine, milk thistle (*Silybum marianum*) is arguably the most highly valued herb for liver support. The extract of milk thistle seeds is primarily made up of silymarin, a mixture of flavonolignans (part flavonoid, part lignan). Silibin is the major component of this mixture. Silibin has been recognized for its ability to benefit people with liver disorders, including hepatitis and cirrhosis.

Various toxins are reduced through the glutathione conjugation pathway, and a deficiency in glutathione can reduce their clearance from the bloodstream. Research has shown that silymarin protects against glutathione depletion and increases liver glutathione status. Since glutathione is one of the primary conjugating agents of phase II, milk thistle can provide significant support to your liver's detoxification mechanism.

Further studies have shown that silymarin may also help prevent the recirculation of toxins and regenerate damaged liver cells. Other studies indicate that milk thistle may prevent liver damage due to liver poisoning from prescription medications. A dosage of 175 mg of milk thistle extract standardized to 80-percent silymarin taken two to three times daily may provide benefits.

It is particularly important to note that some preparations of milk thistle (especially those from China) contain high levels of mycotoxins, which refer to any toxic substance produced by a fungus. As European authorities have standards to ensure the safety of herbal medicines, I would recommend you use milk thistle supplements that contain milk thistle extract from EuroMed or Indena, two pharmaceutical-quality European herbal medicine suppliers that provide herbal extracts to supplement companies. Alternatively, your supplement's label may state that its milk thistle has been tested for mycotoxins, which is also an acceptable way to ensure a product's safety.

Turmeric

Turmeric is a spice commonly used in Asian dishes. It is has also been employed as a therapy in Ayurvedic medicine for many years. The medicinal part of turmeric is its rhizome, the underground stem which looks more like a root due to its thick appearance. In fact, although it is botanically inaccurate, as an herbal medicine this plant is sometimes referred to as "turmeric root." In any case, turmeric's rhizome contains a variety of natural compounds, such as protein, fat, minerals, and carbohydrates. The primary active constituent of raw turmeric is the flavonoid *curcumin,* which is responsible for the turmeric's yellow color and most of its medicinal qualities.

Curcumin contributes to the health of your liver's detoxification system in two ways. First, it encourages the flow of bile, which is beneficial to your digestive functions and promotes the detoxification of environmental and metabolic toxins. Second, curcumin boosts your liver's production of glutathione, which provides antioxidant protection and plays an important role in detoxification via the glutathione conjugation pathway.[26] In regard to its strong antioxidant activity, curcumin has displayed the ability to enhance cellular resistance to oxidative damage.[27] Curcumin has also been found to have hepatoprotective (i.e., liver-protective) properties against a variety of liver-toxic chemicals and drugs.[28] A dosage of 180 to 360 mg of curcumin daily is appropriate.

Supporting the Acetylation Pathway

Conjugation with acetyl-coenzyme A is the primary method by which your body eliminates specific types of drugs, including sulfa drugs. This mechanism, however, appears to be sensitive to genetic variation, as an individual with a poor acetylation system will be far more susceptible to sulfa drugs and other antibiotics. The acetylation pathway includes a type of enzyme called *N-acetyltransferase* (NAT). Genetic defects that affect this enzyme lead to slow metabolism of particular drugs and have been shown to be associated with liver toxicity during certain drug treatments.[29]

Quercetin

Quercetin is a dietary flavonoid that occurs abundantly in red wine, tea, onions, kale, tomatoes, broccoli, green beans, asparagus, apples, and berries.[30] Quercetin has antioxidant, anti-inflammatory, anticarcinogenic, and cardioprotective effects.[31] In one human study, subjects who received supplements of 500 mg of quercetin daily saw their *N-acetyltransferase* activity levels increase by 85 percent on average.[32] This is a good daily dosage.

N-Acetylcysteine

N-acetylcysteine (NAC), previously discussed in association with the sulfation pathway, is an amino acid with, as its name suggests, an acetyl group.[33] As such, it has the potential to support the acetylation pathway. Consistent with this pathway's effect on drugs, NAC has been shown to decrease bladder toxicity caused by the medication ifosfamide.[34] As stated previously, 600 mg is a good daily dosage.

Pantothenic Acid (Vitamin B₅)

Pantothenic acid, also known as vitamin B_5, is required for the metabolism of carbohydrates, proteins, and fats. Pantothenic acid is also a primary precursor of coenzyme A, so named for its role in acetylation reactions.[35] As a precursor to coenzyme A, pantothenic acid plays an important role in supporting the acetylation pathway. A minimum daily dosage of 5 to 10 mg is recommended.

Supporting the Amino Acid Conjugation Pathway

In phase II of detoxification, certain amino acids act as the water-soluble substances to which unwanted molecules are attached. These amino acids include glycine, taurine, glutamine, arginine, and ornithine.[36] Clinically, supplementation with these amino acids has proven to be beneficial for patients with toxic overload, especially when other means of cleansing the body were used at the same time.[37] These amino acids may provide other health benefits as well.

Glycine

A typical diet contains about 2 g of *glycine* daily. The primary source of glycine is protein-rich food, including meat, fish, dairy, and legumes. One of glycine's most significant contributions to human health is the role it plays in promoting healthy liver function. For example, glycine has been shown to prevent liver damage caused by low oxygen levels, reduce mortality due to endotoxin (a toxin that is present inside a bacterial cell and is released when the cell disintegrates), minimize alcoholic liver injury by decreasing blood alcohol levels, and expedite recovery from ethanol-induced liver injury.[38] About 500 to 1,000 mg daily is recommended.

Taurine

Taurine is a compound that is present in high amounts in meat and fish. The most abundant dietary source of taurine, however, is human breast milk. Large amounts of taurine are also found in the human brain, retina, heart, and platelets. Taurine is normally synthesized in the human body in adequate amounts from cysteine and hypotaurine. During prolonged times of insufficient intake, however, the body cannot maintain adequate levels of taurine and supplementation becomes necessary.

Supplementation with additional taurine appears to support the detoxification process. This benefit has been seen in patients with liver or gallbladder disorders who were put on a taurine-supplemented diet. The taurine-supplemented diet increased the concentration of total bile acid in each patient, which indicates that taurine may enhance conjugation and secretion of bile acid and therefore may also boost detoxification.[39] Furthermore, it has been linked to liver health in clinical research in which supplementation with 1.5 to 4 g of taurine daily for up to three months improved liver function in patients with acute and chronic hepatitis as compared to placebo.[40] About 500 to 1,500 mg daily is recommended.

Glutamine

Glutamine is the most abundant amino acid in the human body. It is produced primarily in skeletal muscle and then released into circulation. The parts of your body that require glutamine, such as the immune system, gastrointestinal tract, kidneys, and liver, obtain it as needed from your bloodstream. Glutamine is essential for maintaining intestinal function, immune response, and amino acid homeostasis during times of severe stress.[41] Glutamine is metabolized in your cells' mitochondria and is important for providing metabolic fuel to immune cells such as lymphocytes, macrophages, and fibroblasts.[42] Furthermore, glutamine-containing dipeptides also appear to help preserve intestinal integrity.[43] About 500 to 1,500 mg daily is recommended.

Arginine

Arginine is best known for its beneficial effects on the vascular system. When you take in arginine, your body converts this amino acid into nitric oxide (NO), which causes vasodilation of your blood vessels and thus promotes healthy circulation.[44]

Arginine is also required for the detoxification of ammonia, which is an extremely toxic substance to your central nervous system. Additionally, there is compelling evidence that arginine helps to regulate the functions of multiple organs.[45] Supplementation with arginine has also shown to reduce liver injury in an experimental study.[46] Furthermore, supplementation with 500 to 1,500 mg of arginine seems to reduce some of the symptoms, especially pain, associated with interstitial cystitis (painful bladder syndrome).[47] This is a good daily dosage.

Ornithine

Ornithine is an amino acid produced in the human body from arginine. Research has shown that ornithine can improve some measures of athletic performance.[48] Taking 1 g of ornithine hydrochloride once daily for seven days, and then 3 g with breakfast and lunch immediately before a cycling test was shown to reduce fatigue in healthy volunteers.[49] About 500 to 1,500 mg daily is recommended.

Supporting the Methylation Pathway

The *methylation pathway* involves conjugating methyl groups to toxins in phase II. Support for methylation comes from nutrient cofactors and methyl donors, such as methionine, vitamin B_9 (also known as folate), vitamin B_{12}, vitamin B_6, and betaine.

Methionine

The amino acid *methionine* is one of the primary conjugating compounds involved in methylation. Taking methionine orally seems to be effective in the treatment of acetaminophen poisoning. Supplementation with 2.5 g of methionine every four hours for a total of four doses was shown to be effective in preventing liver damage and death after an acetaminophen overdose when given within ten hours of acetaminophen ingestion.[50] In addition, population research has found that a higher than average dietary intake of methionine is associated with a 6-percent lower risk of breast cancer, especially in post-menopausal women. Increasing dietary intake of methionine by 1 g per day may be associated with a 4-percent reduction in breast cancer risk.[51] About 500 to 1,000 mg daily is recommended.

Vitamin B_9, Vitamin B_{12}, Vitamin B_6

Homocysteine is a byproduct of normal protein metabolism, occurring as part of the methylation process. It is formed from the conversion of the amino acid methionine. As high levels of homocysteine are not a good thing for your health, your body has a built-in mechanism to convert it partially back into methionine and other beneficial amino acids. If, however, this mechanism is not functioning properly, homocysteine can build up in bodily fluids and tissues, leading to serious ramifications.

A substantial body of scientific evidence has shown that vitamin B_9 in the form of folic acid can help lower homocysteine levels.[52] Vitamin B_{12} and vitamin B_6 have also demonstrated similar ability, though each to a lesser extent. To ascertain the lowest dosage of folic acid associated with the maximum reduction in homocysteine concentrations, and to determine the additional relevance of vitamins B_{12} and B_6, the Homocysteine Lowering Trialists' Collaboration conducted a meta-analysis.[53]

According to the results of this meta-analysis, proportional reductions in plasma homocysteine concentrations with folic acid occurred when homocysteine was higher and when folate (folic acid) concentrations were lower before starting therapy. Daily doses of 200 to 800 mcg of folic acid, and some as high as 5 mg, reduced homocysteine levels by 13 to 25 percent. Vitamin B_{12} supplements of 500 mcg per day offered an additional 7-percent reduction in homocysteine levels, but there was a lack of significant effect associated with an average daily dose of 16.5 mg of vitamin B_6. Other research, however, has found that taking vitamin B_6 supplements in combination with folic acid (and sometimes B_{12}) can be effective in lowering homocysteine levels.[54]

A 2004 meta-analysis examining the effectiveness of folic acid in the treatment of depression concluded that the "evidence suggests folate may have a potential role as a supplement to other treatment for depression."[55] Research has also shown that supplementation can lead to an improvement in depressive symptoms.[56] Likewise, patients with celiac disease who were treated with 500 mcg of vitamin B_{12}, 2 mg of vitamin B_6, and 800 mcg of folic acid for six months experienced a drop in homocysteine levels and statistically significant increases in feelings of well-being—notably, improvements in anxiety and depressed mood.[57] Furthermore, folic acid used in conjunction with conventional antidepressants has been shown to improve treatment response.[58] Daily dosage recommendations are 200 to 800 mcg of vitamin B_9, 100 to 500 mcg of vitamin B_{12}, and 10 to 20 mg of vitamin B_6.

Betaine

Not to be confused with betaine hydrochloride, *betaine,* also known as trimethylglycine, or TMG, is a chemical compound that may be useful in certain biochemical reactions in your liver. It is found in such foods as beets, spinach, whole grains, liver, eggs, and seafood. Supplementation with betaine has shown significant reductions in homocysteine levels. Research has shown that a daily dose of 6 g may reduce homocysteine by 15 percent, although significant reductions may also be seen at a dose of 1.5 g daily.[59] About 500 to 1,500 mg daily is recommended.

■ SUPPORTING INTESTINAL DETOXIFICATION

Your gut is one of the most important components of your immune system. Its main role is to absorb nutrients and serve as one of your body's most important barriers. It protects you from potential allergic reactions, as well as microbiological and chemical threats. Your intestines are composed of epithelial cells sitting on your intestinal wall and colonized by trillions of bacteria, which play a role in gut function. In short, your intestinal wall and your friendly bacteria comprise the gut barrier.

Sometimes, however, the gut barrier is compromised. When this happens, the permeability of your intestines' epithelial lining allows the passage of toxins, antigens, and unwanted bacteria to enter your bloodstream. The incidence of impaired and increased intestinal wall permeability, also known as leaky gut syndrome (LGS), is now closely studied because of its potential involvement in many health issues and diseases. Different conditions, such as infection, trauma from burns or surgery, or the use or overuse of many medications, may lead to LGS. These conditions cause inflammation and damage to the intestinal lining. LGS is associated with a wide range of general symptoms, including fatigue, fevers of unknown origin, abdominal pain, bloating and diarrhea, memory problems, concentration difficulties, and poor tolerance to exercise.

Probiotics

Growing evidence shows that your gut microbiota (the sum total of all the bacteria residing in your gut) is important in supporting the epithelial barrier and therefore plays a key role in the regulation of environmental substances that enter the body. Several recent reports have shown that *probiotics,* which refer to live health-promoting bacteria, can help reverse leaky gut by enhancing the production of tight junctions—different types of proteins in the gut barrier that control the flow of molecules in the space between epithelium cells.

Among the various probiotic strains, perhaps the most important issue is stability. The problem is that most probiotics have a relatively short, unstable shelf life, which is why you'll often see many probiotic supplement labels which, after identifying potency (e.g., 1 billion CFU), will include a footnote stating, "at time of manufacture." This, of course, means that by the time a consumer uses a particular probiotic, its actual potency is likely to have diminished.

Unfortunately, this problem is compounded by the fact that, even if stability is adequate on the shelf, many probiotic strains will be destroyed by your stomach acid before they ever reach your gut. If they do reach your intestines, they may be destroyed by bile. Spore-forming probiotic bacteria, however, can overcome these issues, as the spores themselves act as protective encasements, allowing almost indefinite storage until the probiotics are ready to be consumed and ensuring their survival as they travel through the stomach. Examples of spore-forming probiotics include *Bacillus indicus, Bacillus subtilis, Bacillus coagulans, Bacillus licheniformis,* and *Bacillus clausii*. In fact, a combination of these spore-forming probiotics has been studied for its effect on leaky gut.

A thirty-day double-blind placebo-controlled study was conducted to determine if an oral spore-based probiotic supplement could reduce dietary endotoxemia, which is a reflection of toxins that have been absorbed through the intestines and a hallmark of leaky gut syndrome. Seventy-five men and women with apparent endotoxemia received either a placebo (rice flour) or a commercial spore-based probiotic supplement [*Bacillus indicus* (HU36), *Bacillus subtilis* (HU58), *Bacillus coagulans* (SC208), *Bacillus licheniformis,* and *Bacillus clausii*].

The results showed that supplementation with the probiotic blend reduced endotoxins by a significant 42 percent, and also lowered triglycerides by 24 percent. In contrast, the placebo subjects experienced a 36-percent increase in endotoxins and a 5-percent decrease in triglycerides. Furthermore, the spore-forming probiotic supplement was associated with significant reductions in inflammatory markers known as IL-12p70 and IL-1[beta]. The researchers concluded that oral spore-forming probiotic supplementation reduced symptoms indicative of leaky gut syndrome. The recommended daily dosage of each strain is as follows: 1 billion CFU of *Bacillus indicus* (HU36), 2 billion CFU of *Bacillus subtilis* (HU58), 1 billion CFU of *Bacillus coagulans* (SC208), 50 million CFU of *Bacillus licheniformis*, and 1 billion CFU of *Bacillus clausii*.

Prebiotics

Prebiotics can help you maintain a healthy population of friendly bacteria (i.e., probiotics) in your gut and promote a healthy gut barrier so that you may avoid LGS. Prebiotics are generally some type of carbohydrate that serves as nourishment for friendly bacteria, or probiotics, helping them to grow and remain healthy. Acacia gum is one prebiotic that has proven itself successful in achieving this goal in several studies.

Acacia Gum

In one randomized double-blind study, ninety-six healthy volunteers received 6 g of *acacia gum* or 6 g of fructooligosaccharides (FOS)—another type of prebiotic—daily, or 3 g of acacia gum and 3 g of FOS daily. After one week, fecal *Bifidobacteria* increased by seven times in the acacia gum-only group when compared with initial values, and by three times in the FOS-only group. Interestingly, the combination of acacia gum and FOS increased *Bifidobacteria* by almost fourteen times, demonstrating a synergetic effect. In addition, there was a slight reduction in the number of subjects with high counts of *Clostridium perfringens* in those supplementing with acacia gum—which is important, as some strains of *C. perfringens* produce a toxin in the intestine that causes illness.[60]

Another study was conducted in which ten healthy volunteers consumed acacia gum at a dosage of 10 g per day or 15 g per day for ten days, or sucrose as a control. Results showed that concentrations of *Bifidobacteria, Lactobacilli,* and total lactic acid bacteria groups were significantly increased in the acacia gum group at 10 g per day when compared with the control group. This effect on *Bifidobacteria* was even more pronounced (tenfold increase) in subjects who had displayed low initial *Bifidobacteria* counts. This effect was also significant at the dosage of 15 g per day of acacia gum. In addition, the number of weekly stools was slightly increased in the acacia gum groups. Daily stool weight was also higher during acacia gum consumption. These effects may be of interest to people suffering from constipation.[61]

In addition, multiple other studies have demonstrated that acacia gum acts as a prebiotic, increasing the growth of desirable probiotic bacteria.[62] Furthermore, it should be noted that, a few days after it has been ingested, no acacia gum may be found in rat or human feces, meaning that acacia gum is completely broken down by colonic bacteria in the gut and then fermented.[63] As it turns out, this probiotic function has a positive role to play regarding gut barrier function.

In addition to increasing *Bifidobacteria* and *Lactobacilli* counts, acacia gum may also increase the anti-inflammatory bacteria known as *Faecalibacterium prausnitzii*.[64] This likely explains an experiment in which acacia gum reduced pro-inflammatory substances and increased anti-inflammatory substances.[65] As well, samples collected during this experiment were used in a cell line model to study gut wall permeability, the results of which demonstrated that acacia gum seems to enhance the integrity of the intestinal wall.[66] The recommended daily dosage is 5 to10 g.

■ HEAVY METAL DETOXIFICATION

When it comes to the health of their blood, one area of concern for many people is how to go about ridding their systems of heavy metals, especially mercury and lead. The good news is that there are some substances that can help in heavy metal detoxification. These include modified citrus pectin, modified alginate complex, alpha-lipoic acid, N-acetylcysteine, garlic, and selenium.

Modified Citrus Pectin and Modified Alginate Complex

Modified citrus pectin (MCP) is an indigestible complex carbohydrate obtained from the peel and pulp of citrus fruits and processed in such a way as to make it easily absorbed into your bloodstream. Research has shown that 15 g of modified citrus pectin (MCP) daily is capable of reducing (detoxifying) heavy metals in the body.[67] In one study of children, a daily total of 15 g of MCP taken in three divided doses for four weeks resulted in dramatic decreases in blood serum levels of lead (161% average decrease) and dramatic increases in twenty-four-hour urine collection (132% average increase), with no observed adverse effects.[68] When combined with *modified alginate complex* (MAC), another type of complex carbohydrate, the dose of MCP required to reduce heavy metal load may be lessened. Research that utilized 900 to 2,400 mg of MCP combined with 1,350 to 3,600 mg of MAC has shown an associated average decrease in lead and mercury levels of 74 percent.[69] A sufficient daily intake of MCP is approximately 1.5 g, and a sufficient daily intake of MAC is approximately 2.25 g.

Alpha-Lipoic Acid

Inorganic mercury combines with glutathione in your liver and this complex is then secreted in your bile. Consequently, a therapeutic approach that helps increase glutathione levels may be beneficial in cleansing your body of this heavy metal. The antioxidant *alpha-lipoic acid* (ALA) is capable of increasing glutathione status. Furthermore, ALA has been shown to promote the release of glutathione into bile secretions. In animal studies, increases in glutathione levels in bile have been associated with increases in the release of inorganic mercury. ALA given intravenously to rats was shown to boost inorganic mercury release in bile by 1,200 to 4,000 percent immediately after mercury exposure.[70] A daily dosage of 600 mg of ALA is recommended.

N-Acetylcysteine

Research demonstrates that oral administration of N-acetylcysteine, a compound also capable of increasing glutathione levels, produces a profound acceleration of urinary methylmercury excretion in mice.[71] In addition, evidence suggests that the ability of mercury to accumulate in your liver and kidneys might be inversely related to the supply of compounds known as non-protein sulfhydryls in your body. In other words, the more non-protein sulfhydryls you have, the less likely it is for mercury to build up in your system. N-acetylcysteine, a source of these compounds, has shown to be an effective tool against mercury-induced damage to the liver and kidneys, reducing mercury levels in these organs significantly.[72] As such, a daily dosage of 1,200 mg of NAC is recommended in your quest to rid your body of heavy metals.

Garlic Extract

Laboratory research on *garlic extract* suggests that this substance may protect leucocytes, also known as white blood cells, against methylmercury-induced harm.[73] In animal research, garlic has been shown to be protective against methylmercury and phenylmercury poisoning and accumulation in organs, and methylmercury-induced production of certain potentially harmful enzymes.[74] A daily dosage of 1,200 mg of odorless garlic extract or concentrate is recommended.

Selenium

As mentioned in Chapter 4, selenium is an important essential element. The form of selenium known as selenide creates an extremely stable, insoluble compound with mercury, transporting it through membranes for eventual excretion. This action works to lower mercury levels in your body and may provide relief from symptoms of mercury toxicity. Extremely positive results with selenium supplementation were seen in a rural population of 103 villagers in China who had long-term mercury exposure. Subjects were supplemented with 100 mcg of organic selenium daily in the form of selenium-enriched yeast for three months. The results were that organic selenium supplementation effectively increased mercury elimination and decreased urinary levels of two biomarkers of oxidative stress.[75] This dosage of organic selenium is recommended.

CONCLUSION

There are a broad variety of substances that can assist your body in its natural detoxification processes. Daily supplementation with these substances may be followed to provide your body the basic protection it requires against the constant barrage of toxins to which we are all exposed, and at times higher dosages may be employed to promote greater detoxification if necessary. When you take steps to keep your body's overall detoxification system working properly, you also encourage a healthy bloodstream.

9

Complementary Therapies

In addition to diet and dietary supplementation, there are certain complementary therapies that may be used to promote the detoxification process and help you maintain a healthy bloodstream. These therapies are supported by credible research and, in almost every case, should be administered or supervised by a healthcare professional. Therefore, this chapter will review these methods, which include sauna therapy, hydrotherapy, massage therapy, chelation therapy, and meditation, rather than provide instructions on how to participate in them independently.

■ SAUNA THERAPY

Sauna therapy has been shown to provide relief of symptoms that may arise as a result of exposure to toxic environments.[1,2] In the case of those with health problems, however, sauna therapy needs to be carefully tailored to the individual and supervised closely by a healthcare professional.

When you hear the term "sauna," it is typically in reference to the Finnish sauna. The Finnish sauna is a wood-paneled room with wooden benches and a radiant heater that keeps the temperature between 176°F and 194°F at face level, with humidity of 50 to 60 g H_2O vapor/m^3. In sauna therapy, a person sits for two to three sauna sessions of ten to twenty minutes each, which may then be followed by cold immersion.[3]

Saunas have been shown to be an effective preventative measure against certain cardiovascular problems. Their use has proven to reduce blood pressure and enhance blood flow and cardiac function. If using a sauna for its cardiovascular benefits, only short sauna sessions (fifteen minutes) are necessary. Saunas may also be used to enhance the elimination of fat-soluble xenobiotics. For example, cadmium and nickel levels in sweat have been found to be higher than corresponding levels in urine, making perspiration a prime method of detoxification when it comes to cadmium or nickel toxicity.[4] If you would like to use a sauna to mobilize the excretion of heavy metals or other chemical xenobiotics, sessions longer than fifteen minutes will be needed, and these should be medically monitored. For either use, however, sauna therapy can be a safe and practical way to promote blood detoxification and circulation.[5]

■ HYDROTHERAPY

Hydrotherapy, also known as water therapy, aquatic therapy, or pool therapy, refers to the use of water in the treatment of certain health conditions. It has been employed for hundreds of years as part of alternative medicine and is one of the basic methods of treatment still employed by physiotherapists, occupational therapists, and naturopathic medical practitioners. It manipulates water in various ways, including the manipulation of water pressure and temperature, to produce different therapeutic effects on different systems of your body.[6] Modalities of hydrotherapy include the use of water jets, underwater massage, and mineral baths.

Using hydrotherapy in different ways can increase your circulation and boost clearance of your main pathways of detoxification: the skin, kidneys, liver, colon, and lymphatic system. By using water at different temperatures and pressures, you may encourage blood flow and smooth muscle contraction. Hydrotherapy practices also encourage you to incorporate self-care and self-pampering into your daily routine, which can lower blood pressure and promote well-being.

One medical study on the effectiveness of hydrotherapy for detoxification proved it to be effective in the treatment of lead poisoning.[7] This study showed an increase in lead excretion of 250 percent in association with hydrotherapy. In addition, cold-water application in winter swimmers has shown increases in levels of reduced glutathione in red blood cells.[8] Another study demonstrated that wet sheet pack hydrotherapy can produce a statistically significant increase in cognitive function.[9] Other research has shown its usefulness in symptomatic relief of conditions such as rheumatoid arthritis and osteoarthritis, as well as in the management of spasticity.[10,11,12,13]

■ MASSAGE THERAPY

Massage therapy is very beneficial in the treatment of many health conditions. It can help relieve symptoms such as headache, myalgia (muscle pain), and fatigue, and improve the functioning of some organs. In particular, massage improves circulation systemically, which promotes nutritional supply to all tissues, and enhances the removal of toxins from your bloodstream. To achieve these ends, massage movements such as effleurage (circular stroking movement made with the palm of the hand) and petrissage (kneading the body) are applied.

Massage benefits your lymphatic system, increasing the actual flow of lymph in interstitial spaces (i.e., spaces between cells) and promoting the removal of toxins from your body. Stagnation in interstitial spaces can impair lymph flow through the lymph vessels. It can also diminish circulation to tissue cells, slowing their nutritional supply and metabolism. Increasing the flow of lymph with massage therapy benefits your body by delivering nutrients to cells and transporting building materials to restore tissues.[14] Research indicates that massage therapy can create sufficient pressure to push lymph through the gaps between endothelial cells of the collecting lymph vessels. It has also been observed that elevations in the temperature of the skin due to massage therapy can force more junctions between endothelial cells to open. Both of these factors may increase the drainage effect of massage on lymph.[15]

While lymph flow may be enhanced by general strokes for circulation, it can be further aided through the use of more specific techniques, including lymph effleurage and the intermittent pressure technique. You may apply these methods on most regions of your body and alternate them during a therapy session.

Massage can also enhance circulation to specific organs, including the kidneys, liver, and skin. Methods such as compression massage (applying pressure to muscles, which is then held and released) may be used. Massage performed on your entire body as well as locally on your kidney area increases blood flow to and from your kidneys, thereby improving your body's filtration and elimination processes. Systemic lymph massage, as previously noted, leads to a similar outcome. Likewise, your liver is influenced by external pressures, such as those exerted by your diaphragm from above or palpation. With the squeezing movement of massage, enough pressure is exerted through the tissues to influence its circulation.

SITTING VERSUS STANDING

Like most people, you have probably experienced pins and needles in your feet after sitting for an extended period of time. This uncomfortable feeling happens as a result of a reduction in blood circulation in your lower extremities. If you are overweight, sitting for long stretches can negatively affect your circulation to an even greater degree. To support your body's natural detoxification pathways, you need your blood flowing optimally. So, if you spend most of your time in a chair, be sure to take breaks during which you get up and walk around. Taking a walk not only benefits blood flow but also promotes good digestion, both of which work to eliminate harmful substances in your body.

Massage therapy enhances circulation to the liver through the hepatic portal vein. It may also increase the oxygenated blood supply to the liver via the hepatic artery. Massage therapy also boosts circulation along the lobes of the liver, the central and hepatic veins, and the superior vena cava. The mechanical pressure of the massage technique and the resultant increase in blood flow can cause your liver to secrete more bile, which may, in turn, lead to lower blood cholesterol levels. Massage therapy can also increase blood flow to your skin and decongest pores.

■ CHELATION THERAPY

Chelation therapy refers to the binding of metals in your bloodstream to chemical compounds known as "chelators" so that they may be excreted from your body. Chelators bind to metals in a pincer-like fashion (the Greek word "chele" means claw), forming ring-like structures, which are then eliminated through your urine. While chelation therapy can be an important treatment protocol for the removal of toxic metals such as lead and mercury from your bloodstream and tissues, it should be pointed out that chelation may take place naturally as well. For example, relatively weak chelation regularly occurs from eating certain foods such as onions and garlic. Similarly, you may induce chelation by taking certain amino acid supplements orally. That said, the strongest chelation effects occur in association with intravenous chelation therapy, or ICT.

ICT is an FDA–approved treatment for the removal of heavy metals from the body in cases of severe poisoning. In addition, its repeated administration is also used to reduce blood vessel inflammation caused by specific metals and to reduce the body's total load of these metals, especially lead. ICT often utilizes the chelating agent disodium ethylene diamine tetraacetic acid, or EDTA, and, as a result, is sometimes referred to as EDTA chelation.

EDTA chelation has shown the potential to treat atherosclerotic cardiovascular disease, especially heart disease and peripheral artery disease, particularly in diabetics. It has also been proven effective against the progression of nerve damage associated with high blood sugar, also known as diabetic neuropathy. In addition, chelation therapy has been used to treat macular degeneration, osteoporosis, mild to moderate Alzheimer's disease, autoimmune diseases, and fibromyalgia or chronic fatigue syndrome associated with high levels of heavy metals, although less published research exists to support such uses.[16]

Doctors must be well-trained in ICT in order to administer the correct tests and treatments. ICT, however, is not typically taught in conventional medical schools. Rather, it is taught through various professional medical organizations. Perhaps the most recognized leader in educating and certifying healthcare professionals, including MDs and NDs (naturopathic physicians), in chelation therapy is the American College for the Advancement of Medicine (ACAM). ACAM's chelation therapy training teaches doctors how to diagnose and treat patients with heavy metal toxicity as well as how to use diet and nutrients to optimize chelation strategies and protocols.

■ MEDITATION

Similarly to other animals, our ancestors evolved to react to perceived threats to their survival with a specific physiological response known as the flight-or-flight response. Essentially, when you find yourself in immediate danger, your sympathetic nervous system encourages the production of a number of hormones, including cortisol. This reaction is designed to increase your alertness, strength, and speed temporarily, preparing you to flee from an attack or stay and fight it off. While the fight-or-flight response served early humans well by helping to keep them alive in the face of actual life-threatening situations, these days it may do us more harm than good.

Although modern humans don't generally encounter deadly lions or tigers, they do seem to confront a number of psychological stressors in simply trying to make ends meet and get through the week (e.g., traffic jams, overdue bills, work deadlines, abusive employers, school bullies, etc.). Unfortunately, these psychological stressors can set off your fight-or-flight response just as much as physical ones can. Moreover, these psychological stressors are so common that they might have your nervous system working overtime, regularly flooding your bloodstream with hormones that should not be consistently raised. For example, elevations in cortisol, which is also known as the "stress hormone," boost focus and alertness, but they also slow bodily functions such as digestion and detoxification. If your average cortisol level is never allowed to return to its pre-danger reading, then you run the risk of illness.

Meditation practices have proven to be effective at lowering cortisol levels, and regular meditation has been shown to prevent the nervous system from overreacting to stressful situations and keep cortisol at normal levels throughout the day. In addition, by incorporating meditation into your daily routine, you may begin to recognize the value of self-care. This realization may lead you to make better decisions in other aspects of your life, decisions that support a healthy bloodstream and overall body.

CONCLUSION

Each of the complementary therapies discussed in this chapter has value in your quest to eliminate toxins from your bloodstream and body in general. Aside from meditation, however, each one of these therapies requires a healthcare professional to administer it properly, or at least to oversee the process. In the case of ICT, of course, a licensed physician (MD, DO, or ND) must administer the therapy. In the case of massage, a qualified massage therapist can do the job nicely. Hydrotherapy is probably best administered by an ND, since NDs are trained in this modality. While access to a sauna may be gained without a healthcare professional, it is best to consult with one to determine the length and frequency of your sauna sessions. Whether you try one or all of these options, merely taking the time to concentrate on caring for yourself may lead you to alter the way you approach your life for the better, which may then lead to positive health outcomes in general.

Conclusion

Now that you have taken in all the useful information provided by this book, one question remains: How do you incorporate what you now know into your daily life? It is one thing to understand what needs to be done in order to support healthy blood; it is quite another to do it. The first step in adopting these lifestyle changes is realizing why you are adopting them. Your reason for choosing certain foods and engaging in particular activities isn't merely to experience the satisfaction of seeing what you've been told are good numbers on a blood test. Your reason for changing your routine is to avoid potential health problems such as heart disease, cancer, stroke, and type 2 diabetes.

If you provide your body with what it needs to function optimally, its natural pathways of detoxification and cleansing will eliminate unwanted substances from your blood—substances that have been linked to the conditions previously mentioned. In other words, you have the ability to take a significant degree of control over your well-being. By knowing what's in your blood and what you should do about it, you no longer need to feel like a passenger in your own life, forced to go where your genetics take you. This book is designed to help you put your hands on the wheel and steer yourself towards a healthier, happier life.

You now understand why you should follow the advice in this book and change your habits. What you may not yet understand is that how to do so isn't as difficult as you might think. When putting food on your plate, choose predominantly whole grains, non-starchy vegetables, fruit, legumes, and nuts. Opting for a mainly plant-based diet and significantly reducing your red meat consumption will go a long way in keeping your bloodstream at its best. If you use beneficial herbs and spices to season your meals and cook them using techniques that will ensure they contain the maximum amount of nutrients, your food will help the state of your blood even more.

Aside from watching your diet, learning how to breathe better is important, as doing so increases your oxygen levels and thus improves the health of your blood. Thankfully, you can breathe better simply by improving your posture, laughing more, and meditating. Even massage can be helpful, as it facilitates the movement of oxygen-rich blood to the tissues that need it.

Finally, you may use certain supplements to support your body's natural pathways of detoxification, or even try complementary therapies such as sauna therapy, hydrotherapy, or, as recently mentioned, massage therapy, which may promote the detoxification process and a healthy bloodstream.

Your blood is the primary means of transport for both the helpful and the harmful substances inside your body. It is the common denominator of your well-being. The fact that you have a considerable amount of influence on your blood means you have a remarkable degree of power over your own health. Fortunately, you have at your fingertips all the information you require to make your influence a positive one.

References

Chapter 1

1. Betts J.G., Desaix P., Johnson E., et al. *Anatomy & Physiology*. Houston, TX: OpenStax, 2013.

2. Maton, A., Hopkins, J., McLaughlin, C. W., Susan J., Warner, M. Q., LaHart, D., and J. D. Wright. *Human Biology and Health*. Englewood Cliffs, New Jersey: Prentice Hall, 1993.

3. Alberts B., Johnson, A., Lewis, J., Raff, M., Roberts, K., and P. Walter. *Molecular Biology of the Cell*. 4th Ed. New York: Garland Science, 2002.

4. Doan, Charles A. "The White Blood Cells in Health and Disease." *Bull NY Acad Med* 30, 6 (Jun. 1954): 415–428.

5. Laki, K. "Our ancient heritage in blood clotting and some of its consequences." *Ann NY Acad Sci* 202 (Dec. 8, 1972): 297–307.

6. Abelow, B. *Understanding Acid-Base*. New York: Lippincott Williams & Wilkins, 1998.

7. Garrett, R. H., and C. M. Grisham. *Biochemistry*. Boston: Cengage Learning, 2010.

8. Xu L., and I. J. Fidler. "Acidic pH-induced elevation in interleukin 8 expression by human ovarian carcinoma cells." *Cancer Research* 60, 16 (Aug. 15, 2000): 4610–4616.

9. Rafiee, P., Nelson, V. M., Manley, S., Wellner, M., Floer, M., Binion, D. G., and R. Shaker. "Effect of curcumin on acidic pH-induced expression of IL-6 and IL-8 in human esophageal epithelial cells (HET-1A): role of PKC, MAPKs, and NF-kappaB." *Am J Physiol Gastrointest Liver Physiol* 296 (2009): G388–G398.

10. Krieger, N. S., Sessler, N. E., and D. A. Bushinsky. "Acidosis inhibits osteoblastic and stimulates osteoclastic activity in vitro." *Am J Physiol* 262, 3 Pt 2 (Mar. 1992): F442–F448.

11. Arnett, T. R., and D. W. Dempster. "Effect of pH on bone resorption by rat osteoclasts in vitro." *Endocrinology* 119, 1 (Jul. 1986): 119–124.

12. Arnett, T. R., and M. Spowage. "Modulation of the resorptive activity of rat osteoclasts by small changes in extracellular pH near the physiological range." *Bone* 18, 3 (Mar. 1996): 277–279.

13. Grinspoon, S. K., Baum, H. B., Kim, V., Coggins, C., and A. Klibanski. "Decreased bone formation and increased mineral dissolution during acute fasting in young women." *J Clin Endocrinol Metab* 80, 12 (Dec. 1995): 3628–3633.

14. U.S. Department of Agriculture and U.S. Department of Health and Human Services. *Dietary Guidelines for Americans, 2010.* 7th Edition. Washington, D.C.: U.S. Government Printing Office, December 2010.

15. "Report Card on the Quality of Americans' Diets." *Nutrition Insights* Insight 28. USDA Center for Nutrition Policy and Promotion, December 2002.

16. "Diet Quality of Americans in 2001–02 and 2007–08 as Measured by the Healthy Eating Index-2010." Nutrition Insight 51. USDA Center for Nutrition Policy and Promotion, April 2013.

17. Frassetto, L., Morris, R. C. Jr., Sellmeyer, D. E., Todd, K., and A. Sebastian. "Diet, evolution and aging: The pathophysiologic effects of the post-agricultural inversion of the potassium-to-sodium and base-to-chloride ratios in the human diet." *Eur J Nutr* 40 (2001): 200–213.

18. Schwalfenberg, G. K. "The Alkaline Diet: Is There Evidence That an Alkaline pH Diet Benefits Health?" *Journal of Environmental and Public Health* Volume 2012, Article ID 727630, 7 pages: doi:10.1155/2012/727630.

19. Centers for Disease Control and Prevention. "Physical Activity Facts." cdc. gov. https://www.cdc.gov/healthyschools/physicalactivity/facts.htm (accessed Apr. 9, 2018).

20. Myers J. "Exercise and Cardiovascular Health." *Circulation* 107, 1 (2003): e2–e5.

21 Ibid.

22. United States Environmental Protection Agency. "2010 Toxics Release Inventory National Analysis Overview." epa.gov. https://www.epa.gov/sites/production/files/documents/2010_national_analysis_overview_document.pdf (accessed Jan. 17, 2016).

23. Ashford, N., and C. Miller. *Chemical Exposures: Low Levels and High Stakes.* 2nd Ed. New York: John Wiley & Sons, Inc.,1998.

24. Terr, A. "Environmental Illness: A Clinical Review of 50 Cases." *Arch Intern Med* 146, 1 (Jan. 1986): 145–149.

25. Lawson, L. *Staying Well in a Toxic World.* Chicago: The Nobel Press, Inc., 1993.

26. Shin, S., Fauman, E. B., Petersen, A., et al. "An atlas of genetic influences on human blood metabolites." *Nature Genetics* 46 (2014): 543–550.

27. National Heart, Lung, and Blood Institute. "Sickle Cell Disease." nhlbi.nih. gov. https://www.nhlbi.nih.gov/health-topics/sickle-cell-disease (accessed Aug. 2, 2016).

28. Starr, P. S. "Genetic blood disorders: Questions you need to ask." *J Fam Pract* 61, 1 (Jan. 2012): 30–37.

29. Ibid.

30. Ibid.

31. Ibid.

32. Mayo Clinic. "Leukemia: Risk factors." mayoclinic.org. http://www.mayoclinic .org/diseases-conditions/leukemia/basics/risk-factors/con-20024914 (accessed Jan. 17, 2017).

33. Carey, N. *Epigenetics Revolution: How Modern Biology Is Rewriting Our Understanding of Genetics, Disease and Inheritance.* London: Icon Books, 2011.

34. Betts J.G., Desaix P., Johnson E., et al. *Anatomy & Physiology.* Houston, TX: OpenStax, 2013.

35. Ibid.

36. Ibid.

37. Ibid.

38. Ibid.

39. Ibid.

Chapter 2

1. LaValle J. B. *Your Blood Never Lies: How to Read a Blood Test for a Longer, Healthier Life.* Garden City Park, NY: Square One Publishers, 2013.

2. U.S. Department of Health and Human Services and U.S. Department of Agriculture. "Dietary Guidelines for Americans 2015–2020. Eighth Edition." health.gov. http://health.gov/dietaryguidelines/2015/guidelines (accessed Jan. 8, 2016).

3. U.S. Department of Agriculture Agricultural Research Service. "What We Eat in America, NHANES 2011–2012." ars.usda.gov. http://www.ars.usda.gov/ SP2UserFiles/Place/80400530/pdf/1112/tables_1-40_2011-2012.pdf (accessed Jan. 8, 2016).

4. Roger, V. L., Go, A. S., Lloyd-Jones, D. M., Adams, R. J., Berry, J. D., Brown, T. M., et al. "Heart disease and stroke statistics—2011 update: a report from the American Heart Association." *Circulation* 123, 4 (Feb. 2011): e18–e209.

5. Danaei, G., Ding, E. L., Mozaffarian, D., Taylor, B., Rehm, J., Murray, C. J., et al. "The preventable causes of death in the United States: comparative risk assessment of dietary, lifestyle, and metabolic risk factors." *PLoS Med* 6, 4 (Apr. 28, 2009): e1000058.

6. Stampfer, M. J., Malinow, R., Willett, W. C., et al. "A prospective study of plasma homocyst(e)ine and risk of myocardial infarction in US physicians." *JAMA* 268, 7 (Aug. 19, 1992): 877–881.

7. Bostom, A. G., Silbershatz, H., Rosenberg, I. H., et al. "Nonfasting plasma total

homocysteine levels and all-cause and cardiovascular disease mortality in elderly Framingham men and women." *Arch Intern Med* 159, 10 (May 24, 1999):1077–1080.

8. Tiemeier, H., van Tuijl, H. R., Hofman, A., et al. "Vitamin B12, folate, and homocysteine in depression: the Rotterdam study." *Am J Psychiatry* 159, 12 (Dec 2002): 2099–2101.

9. Regland, B., Andersson, M., Abrahamsson, L., et al. "Increased concentrations of homocysteine in the cerebrospinal fluid in patients with fibromyalgia and chronic fatigue syndrome." *Scand J Rheumatol* 26, 4 (1997): 301–307.

10. Ho, R. C., Cheung, M. W., Fu, E., Win, H. H., Zaw, M. H., Ng, A., and A. Mak. "Is high homocysteine level a risk factor for cognitive decline in elderly? A systematic review, meta-analysis, and meta-regression." *Am J Geriatr Psychiatry* 19, 7 (Jul. 2011): 607–617.

Chapter 3

1. Rutter, M., and R. Russell-Jones, eds. Lead versus Health: Sources and Effects of Low Level Lead Exposure. Chichester, NY: John Wiley & Sons, 1983.

2. Yost, K. J. "Cadmium, the environment and human health. An overview." *Experentia* 40 (1984): 157–164.

3. Gerstner, B. G., and J. E. Huff. "Clinical toxicology of mercury." *J Toxicol Environ Health* 2, 3 (Jan. 1977): 471–526.

4. Nation, J. R., Hare, M. F., Baker, D. M., et al. "Dietary administration of nickel: effects on behavior and metallothionein levels." *Physiol Behavior* 34, 3 (Mar. 1985): 349–353.

5. Editorial. "Toxicologic consequences of oral aluminum." *Nutr Rev* 45 (1987): 72–74.

6. Passwater, R. A., and E. M. Cranton. *Trace Elements, Hair Analysis and Nutrition.* New Canaan, CT: Keats, 1983.

7. Pizzorno J. E. Jr., and M. T. Murray. *Textbook of Natural Medicine.* Second Edition. Edinburgh: Churchill Livingstone, 1999.

8. Hunter, B. "Some food additives as neuroexcitors and neurotoxins." *Clinical Ecology* 2 (1984): 83–89.

9. Cullen, M. R. *Workers with Multiple Chemical Sensitivities: Occupational Medicine State of the Art Reviews.* Philadelphia, PA: Hanley & Belfus, 1987.

10. Stayner, L. T., Elliott, L., Blade, L., et al. "A retrospective cohort mortality study of workers exposed to formaldehyde in the garment industry." *Am J Ind Med* 13, 6 (1988): 667–681.

11. Kilburn, K. H., Warshaw, R., Boylen, C. T., et al. "Pulmonary and neurobehavioral effects of formaldehyde exposure." *Archiv Environ Health* 40, 5 (Sep. 1985): 254–260.

12. Sterling, T. D., and A. V. Arundel. "Health effects of phenoxy herbicides." *Scand J Work Environ Health* 12, 3 (Jun. 1986): 161–173.

13. Dickey L. D., Ed. *Clinical Ecology.* Springfield, IL: CC Thomas, 1976.

14. Lindstrom, K., Riihimaki, H., and K. Hannininen. "Occupational solvent exposure and neuropsychiatric disorders." *Scan J Work Environ Health* 10, 5 (Oct. 1984): 321–323.

15. Pizzorno J. E. Jr., and M. T. Murray. *Textbook of Natural Medicine.* Second Edition. Edinburgh: Churchill Livingstone, 1999.

16. Ibid.

17. Murray, R. K., Granner, D. K., Mayes, P. A., and V. W. Rodwell. *Harper's Biochemistry.* 25th Ed. New York: McGraw Hill, 2000.

18. Lüllmann H., Mohr, K., Ziegler, A., and D. Bieger. *Color Atlas of Pharmacology.* 2nd Ed. Stuttgart: Thieme, 2000.

19. Roundtree, R. "The Use of Phytochemicals in the Biotransformation and Elimination of Environmental Toxins." In *Medicines from the Earth 2003: Official Proceedings,* 115–128. Brevard, North Carolina: Gaia Herbal Research Institute, 2003.

20. Murray, R. K., Granner, D. K., Mayes, P. A., and V. W. Rodwell. *Harper's Biochemistry.* 25th Ed. New York: McGraw Hill, 2000.

21. Lüllmann H., Mohr, K., Ziegler, A., and D. Bieger. *Color Atlas of Pharmacology.* 2nd Ed. Stuttgart: Thieme, 2000.

22. Murray, R. K., Granner, D. K., Mayes, P. A., and V. W. Rodwell. *Harper's Biochemistry.* 25th Ed. New York: McGraw Hill, 2000.

23. Lüllmann H., Mohr, K., Ziegler, A., and D. Bieger. *Color Atlas of Pharmacology.* 2nd Ed. Stuttgart: Thieme, 2000.

24. Pacifici, G. M., Viani, A., Franch, M., Santerini, S., Temellini, A., Giuliani, L., and M. Carra. "Conjugation pathways in liver disease." *Br J Clin Pharmac* 30 (1990): 427–435.

25. Liska, D. J. "The detoxification enzyme systems." *Altern Med Rev* 3, 3 (Jun. 1998):187–198.

26. Murray, R. K., Granner, D. K., Mayes, P. A., and V. W. Rodwell. *Harper's Biochemistry.* 25th Ed. New York: McGraw Hill, 2000.

27. Jakoby, W. B., and D. M. Ziegler. "The enzymes of detoxication." *J Biol Chem* 265, 34 (Dec. 5, 1990) 265, 34: 20715–20718.

28. Liska D, Lynon M, Jones DS. Detoxification and Biotransformational Imbalances. In *Textbook of Functional Medicine,* edited by David S. Jones, 275–298. Gig Harbor, WA: Institute for Functional Medicine; 2006.

29. Liska, D. J. "The detoxification enzyme systems." *Altern Med Rev* 3, 3 (Jun. 1998):187–198.

30. Carey, W. D. *Current Clinical Medicine.* 2nd Ed. Philadelphia: Elsevier, 2010.

31. Ueda, K., Clark, D. P., Chen, C. J., et al. "The human multidrug resistance (mdr1) gene. cDNA cloning and transcription initiation." *J Biol Chem* 262, 2 (Jan. 1987): 505–508.

32. Shade, C. "Mercury and the human detoxification system." Klinghardt

Academy. Sep. 11, 2010. http://www.klinghardtacademy.com/images/stories/powerpoints/microsilica%202009.pdf.

33. Pizzorno J. E. Jr., and M. T. Murray. *Textbook of Natural Medicine*. Second Edition. Edinburgh: Churchill Livingstone, 1999.

Chapter 4

1. Whitney, E., and R. R. Rolfes. *Understanding Nutrition*. 11th ed. Belmont, CA: Thompson Learning, 2008.

2. Ibid.

3. Ibid.

4. Ibid.

5. Ibid.

6. Ibid.

Chapter 5

1. Whitney, E., and R. R. Rolfes. *Understanding Nutrition*. 11th Ed. Belmont, CA: Thompson Learning, 2008.

2. Ibid.

3. Bazzano, L. A. "Effects of soluble dietary fiber on low-density lipoprotein cholesterol and coronary heart disease risk." *Curr Atheroscler Rep* 10, 6 (Dec. 2008): 473–477.

4. O'Keefe, J. H., Gheewala, N. M., and J. O. O'Keefe. "Dietary strategies for improving post-prandial glucose, lipids, inflammation, and cardiovascular health." *J Am Coll Cardiol* 51, 3 (Jan. 22, 2008): 249–55.

5. Ibid.

6. Jacobs, D. R. Jr., Marquart, L., Slavin, J., and L. H. Kushi. "Whole grain intake and cancer: an expanded review and meta-analysis." *Nutrition and Cancer* 30, 2 (1998): 85–90.

7. Chatenoud, L., Tavani, A., La Vecchia, C., et al. "Whole grain intake and cancer risk." *Int J Cancer* 77, 1 (Jul. 3, 1998): 24–28.

8. World Cancer Research Fund / American Institute for Cancer Research. Food, Nutrition, Physical Activity, and the Prevention of Cancer: a Global Perspective. Washington, DC: AICR, 2007.

9. Ibid.

10. Rungapamestry, V., Duncan, A. J., Fuller, Z., and B. Ratcliffe. "Effect of cooking brassica vegetables on the subsequent hydrolysis and metabolic fate of glucosinolates." *Proc Nutr Soc* 66, 1 (Feb. 2007): 69–81.

11. Volden, J., Borge, G. I. A., Bengtsson, G. B., Hansen, M., Thygesen, I. E., and T. Wicklund. "Effect of thermal treatment on glucosinolates and antioxidant-related parameters in red cabbage (*Brassica oleracea* L. ssp. *capitata* f. *rubra*)." *Food Chemistry* 109, 3 (Aug. 2008): 595–605.

12. Whitney, E., and R. R. Rolfes. *Understanding Nutrition.* 11th Ed. Belmont, CA: Thompson Learning, 2008.

13. Spence, J. D. "Stroke prevention in the high-risk patient." *Expert Opin Pharmacother* 8, 12 (Aug. 2007): 1851–1859.

14. Mayo Clinic. "Mediterranean diet: a heart-healthy eating plan." mayoclinic. org. https://www.mayoclinic.org/healthy-lifestyle/nutrition-and-healthy-eating/in-depth/mediterranean-diet/art-20047801 (accessed Jan. 21, 2018).

15. Ibid.

16. Willett, W. C., and M. J. Stampfer. "Rebuilding the food pyramid." Scientific American 288, 1 (Jan. 2003): 66–67.

17. Whitney, E., and R. R. Rolfes. *Understanding Nutrition.* 11th Ed. Belmont, CA: Thompson Learning, 2008.

18. O'Keefe, J. H., Gheewala, N. M., and J. O. O'Keefe. "Dietary strategies for improving post-prandial glucose, lipids, inflammation, and cardiovascular health." *J Am Coll Cardiol* 51, 3 (Jan. 22, 2008): 249–55.

19. Sartorelli, D. S., and M. A. Cardoso. "[Association between dietary carbohydrates and type 2 diabetes mellitus: epidemiological evidence.]" *Arq Bras Endocrinol Metabol* 50, 3 (Jun. 2006): 415–426.

20. U.S. Department of Agriculture. "All About the Grains Group." choosemyplate.gov. https://www.choosemyplate.gov/grains (accessed Mar. 8, 2017).

21. Benzie, I. F., and S. W. Choi. "Antioxidants in food: content, measurement, significance, action, cautions, caveats, and research needs." *Adv Food Nutr Res* 71 (2014): 1–53.

22. U.S. Department of Agriculture Agricultural Research Service. "USDA Food Composition Databases." nal.usda.gov. https://ndb.nal.usda.gov/ndb (accessed Apr. 12, 2018).

23. Ibid.

24. Ibid.

25. U.S. Department of Agriculture. "All About the Fruit Group." choosemyplate. gov. https://www.choosemyplate.gov/fruit (accessed Mar. 8, 2017).

26. Benzie, I. F., and S. W. Choi. "Antioxidants in food: content, measurement, significance, action, cautions, caveats, and research needs." *Adv Food Nutr Res* 71 (2014): 1–53.

27. U.S. Department of Agriculture. "All About the Vegetable Group." choosemyplate.gov. https://www.choosemyplate.gov/vegetables (accessed Mar. 8, 2017).

28. U.S. Department of Agriculture. "All About the Protein Foods Group." choosemyplate.gov. https://www.choosemyplate.gov/protein-foods (accessed Mar. 8, 2017).

29. American Heart Association. "Meat, Poultry, and Fish: Picking Healthy

Proteins." heart.org. https://healthyforgood.heart.org/eat-smart/articles/meat-poultry-and-fish-picking-healthy-proteins (accessed Nov. 11, 2017).

30. SELFNutritionData. "Chickpeas (garbanzo beans, bengal gram), mature seeds, cooked, boiled, without salt. Nutrition Facts & Calories." self.com. http://nutritiondata.self.com/facts/legumes-and-legume-products/4326/2 (accessed Mar. 8, 2018).

31. Birt, D. F., Boylston, T., Hendrich, S., et al. "Resistant starch: promise for improving human health." *Advances in Nutrition* 4, 6 (Nov. 6, 2013): 587–601.

32. Sabaté J., Wien, M. "A perspective on vegetarian dietary patterns and risk of metabolic syndrome." *British Journal of Nutrition* 113, Suppl 2 (Apr. 2015): S136–43.

33. Young, L. "Benefits of Nuts and Seeds: 7 Winners." huffpost.com. https://www.huffpost.com/entry/healthy-foods_b_2115225 (accessed Mar. 12, 2018).

34. Massachusetts Department of Public Health. "Mass in Motion: Eating Better and Moving More." mass.gov. https://www.mass.gov/mass-in-motion-eating-better-and-moving-more (accessed Mar. 12, 2018).

35. National Institutes of Health. "The Surgeon General's Report on Bone Health and Osteoporosis: What It Means to You." bones.nih.gov. https://www.bones.nih.gov/health-info/bone/SGR/surgeon-generals-report (accessed Dec. 1, 2017).

36. National Institutes of Health National Heart, Lung, and Blood Institute. "Your Guide to Lowering Your Blood Pressure With DASH." NIH Publication No. 06-4082. https://www.nhlbi.nih.gov/files/docs/public/heart/new_dash.pdf (accessed Dec. 1, 2017).

37. U.S. Department of Agriculture National Agricultural Library. "Organic Production/ Organic Food: Information Access Tools." nal.usda.gov. https://www.nal.usda.gov/afsic/organic-productionorganic-food-information-access-tools (accessed Dec. 1, 2017).

38. Kristensen, E. S. "Food safety in an organic perspective." 14th IFOAM Congress, Victoria, Canada. August 22nd 2002. http://orgprints.org/19/03/Kristensen_IFOAM_2002.ppt (accessed May 25, 2005).

39. Ibid.

40. Magkos, F., Arvaniti, F., and A. Zampelas. "Organic food: nutritious food or food for thought? A review of the evidence." *Int J Food Sci Nutr* 54, 5 (Sep. 2003): 357–371.

41. U.S. Department of Agriculture Agricultural Research Service. "USDA Food Composition Databases." nal.usda.gov. https://ndb.nal.usda.gov/ndb (accessed Apr. 12, 2018).

42. Holmboe-Ottesen, G. "[Better health with ecologic food?]" *Tidsskrift Nor Laegeforen* 124, 11 (Jun. 3, 2004):1529–1531.

43. U.S. Department of Agriculture Agricultural Research Service. "USDA Food Composition Databases." nal.usda.gov. https://ndb.nal.usda.gov/ndb (accessed Apr. 12, 2018).

44. Ibid.

45. Ibid.

46. Ibid.

47. Magkos, F., Arvaniti, F., and A. Zampelas. "Organic food: nutritious food or food for thought? A review of the evidence." *Int J Food Sci Nutr* 54, 5 (Sep. 2003): 357–371.

48. U.S. Department of Agriculture Agricultural Research Service. "USDA Food Composition Databases." nal.usda.gov. https://ndb.nal.usda.gov/ndb (accessed Apr. 12, 2018).

49 Ibid.

50. Ibid.

51. Holmboe-Ottesen, G. "[Better health with ecologic food?]" *Tidsskrift Nor Laegeforen* 124, 11 (Jun. 3, 2004):1529–1531.

52. Atkins R. C. *Dr. Atkins New Diet Revolution.* New York: Quill, 2002.

53. Brehm, B. J., Seeley, R. J., Daniels, S. R., et al. "A randomized trial comparing a very low carbohydrate diet and a calorie-restricted low fat diet on body weight and cardiovascular risk factors in healthy women." *J Clin Endocrinol Metab* 88, 4 (Apr. 2003): 1617–1623.

54. Foster, G. D., Wyatt, H. R., Hill, J.O., et al. "A randomized trial of a low-carbohydrate diet for obesity." *N Engl J Med* 348, 21 (May 22, 2003): 2082–2090.

55. Walker, C., and B. V. Reamy. "Diets for cardiovascular disease prevention: what is the evidence?" *Am Fam Physician* 79, 7 (Apr. 1, 2009): 571–578.

56. Mente, A., de Koning, L., Shannon, H. S., and S. S. Anand. "A systematic review of the evidence supporting a causal link between dietary factors and coronary heart disease." *Arch Intern Med* 169, 7 (Apr. 13, 2009): 659–69.

57. Shai, I., Schwarzfuchs, D., Henkin, Y., et al. "Weight loss with a low-carbohydrate, Mediterranean, or low-fat diet." *N Engl J Med* 359, 3 (Jul. 17, 2008): 229--241.

58 Krebs-Smith, S. M., and P. Kris-Etherton. "How does MyPyramid compare to other population-based recommendations for controlling chronic disease?" *J Am Diet Assoc* 107, 5 (May 2007): 830–837.

59. Ibid.

60. Douglass, J. M. "Raw diet and insulin requirements." *Ann Intern Med* 82, 1 (Jan. 1975): 61–62.

61. Fontana, L., Meyer, T. E., Klein, S., and J. O. Holloszy. "Long-term low-calorie low-protein vegan diet and endurance exercise are associated with low cardiometabolic risk." *Rejuvenation Res* 10, 2 (Jun. 2007): 225–234.

62. Key, T. J., Thorogood, M., Appleby, P. N., and M. L. Burr. "Dietary habits and mortality in 11,000 vegetarians and health conscious people: results of a 17 year follow up." *BMJ* 313, 7060 (Sep. 28, 1996): 775–779.

63. Link, L. B., Hussaini, N. S., and J. S. Jacobson. "Change in quality of life and

immune markers after a stay at a raw vegan institute: a pilot study." *Complement Ther Med* 16, 3 (Jun. 2008): 124–130.

Chapter 6

1. Jensen, F. B. "The dual roles of red blood cells in tissue oxygen delivery: oxygen carriers and regulators of local blood flow." *J Exp Biol* 212, Pt 21 (Nov. 2009): 3387–3393.

2. Gibney, M. J., Lanham-New, S. A., Cassidy, A., and H. H. Vorster (Eds.). *Introduction to Human Nutrition.* 2nd Edition. West Sussex, UK: Wiley-Blackwell, 2009.

3. Pham-Huy, L. A., He, H., and C. Pham-Huy. "Free radicals, antioxidants in disease and health." *Int J Biomed Sci* 4, 2 (Jun. 2008): 89–96.

4. Florence, T. M. "The role of free radicals in disease." *Aust N Z J Ophthalmol* 23, 1 (Feb. 1995): 3–7.

5. Pham-Huy, L. A., He, H., and C. Pham-Huy. "Free radicals, antioxidants in disease and health." *Int J Biomed Sci* 4, 2 (Jun. 2008): 89–96.

6. Alaska Department of Health and Social Services, Division of Public Health, Section of Injury Prevention and EMS. "Chapter 4: Hypoxia and Oxygenation." In *Alaska Air Medical Escort Training Manual.* 4th Ed. Juneau, AK: Alaska Department of Health and Social Services, 2006.

7. Ibid.

8. Ibid.

9. Pathway Medicine. "Carbon Monoxide and Oxygen Transport." pathwaymedicine.org. http://www.pathwaymedicine.org/carbon-monoxide-and-oxygen-transport (accessed Jan. 18, 2018).

10. Siddiqui, A. "Effects of vasodilation and arterial resistance on cardiac output." *J Clinic Experiment Cardiol* 2 (Dec. 20, 2011):170.

11. Quastel, J. H. "Biochemical effects of administration of narcotics and alcohol." In *Origins of Resistance to Toxic Agents: Proceedings of the Symposium held in Washington, D.C., March 25–27, 1954* edited by Sevag M. G., Reid R. D., and R. E. Reynolds, 209–222. New York: Academic Press, 1955.

12. Sircus, M. *Anti-Inflammatory Oxygen Therapy.* Garden City Park, NY: Square One Publishers, 2015.

Chapter 7

1. Jeffrey, E. H. "Diet and Detoxification Enzymes." *The Proceedings from the 13th International Symposium of The Institute for Functional Medicine.* Supplement to *Alternative Therapies in Health and Medicine.* 2009: S98–S99.

2. Jones, W. *Cure Constipation.* Now. New York: Berkley Publishing Group; 2009.

3. Web MD. 2005–2011. "The Basics of Constipation." Accessed April 19, 2011 http://www.webmd.com/digestive-disorders/digestive-diseases-constipation.

4. National Center for Health Statistics. "Dietary Intake of Macronutrients, Micronutrients, and Other Dietary Constituents: United States, 1988–94." *Vital and Health Statistics* Series 11, Number 245. July, 2002.

5. Institute of Medicine. "Dietary, Functional, and Total Fiber. Dietary Reference Intakes for Energy, Carbohydrate, Fiber, Fat, Fatty Acids, Cholesterol, Protein, and Amino Acids." Washington, D. C.: National Academies Press, 2002: 265–334.

6. The National Digestive Diseases Information Clearinghouse, a service of the National Institute of Diabetes and Digestive and Kidney Diseases. "Constipation." NIH Publication No. 07–2754. July 2007. Accessed April 19, 2011 http://digestive. niddk.nih.gov/ddiseases/pubs/constipation/#serious.

7. Ibid.

8. Williams, E. W., Hemmings, W. A. "Intestinal uptake and transport of proteins in the adult rat." *Proc R Soc London Br* 203 (1979): 177–189.

9. Warshaw, A. L., Bellini C. A., Walker W. A. "The intestinal mucosal barrier to intact antigenic protein." *Am J Surg* 133 (1977): 55–58.

10 Khalif, I. L., Quigley, E. M., Konovitch, E. A, Maximova, I. D. "Alterations in the colonic flora and intestinal permeability and evidence of immune activation in chronic constipation." *Dig Liver Dis*. 37, 11 (2005): 838–849.

11. Friend, B. A., Shahani, K. M. "Nutritional and therapeutic aspects of lactobacilli." *J App Nutr* 36 (1984):125–136.

12. Reddy, B. S. "Dietary fat and its relationship to large bowel cancer." *Cancer Res* 41 (1981): 3700–3705.

13. Mills, S. *The Essential Book of Herbal Medicine*. London: Arkana/Penguin, 1991.

14. Jeffery, E. H. "Diet and Detoxification Enzymes." *The Proceedings from the 13th International Symposium of The Institute for Functional Medicine*. Supplement to *Alternative Therapies in Health and Medicine* 2009: S98–S99.

15. Saito, M., Hirata-Koizumi, M., Matsumoto, M., Urano, T., Hasegawa, R. "Undesirable effects of citrus juice on the pharmacokinetics of drugs: focus on recent studies." *Drug Safety* 28, 8 (2005): 677–694.

16. Foroutan, R. "What's the Deal with Detox Diets? Eat Right, Academy of Nutrition and Dietetics." Published April 26, 2017. Reviewed March 2018. Retrieved June 3, 2018 from https://www.eatright.org/health/weight-loss/ fad-diets/whats-the-deal-with-detox-diets.

17. Marlett, J. A., McBurney, M. I., Slavin, J. L. "Position of the American Dietetic Association: health implications of dietary fiber." *J Am Diet Assoc* 102, 7 (2002): 993–1000.

18. Cummings, J.H. "The effect of dietary fiber on fecal weight and composition." In: Spiller GA, ed. *Fiber in Human Nutrition*. 3rd ed. Boca Raton: CRC Press; 2001.

19. Anti, M., Pignataro, G., Armuzzi, A., et al. "Water supplementation enhances the effect of high-fiber diet on stool frequency and laxative consumption in adult patients with functional constipation." *Hepatogastroenterology*. 45, 21 (1998): 727–732.

20. American Academy of Family Physicians. "Constipation: Keeping Your Bowels Moving Smoothly [Web page]". April 2000. Available at: http://familydoctor.org/ online/famdocen/home/common/digestive/basics/037. html. Accessed September 14, 2004.

21. WebMD. 2005–2011. "Exercise to Ease Constipation." Retrieved April 19, 2011 from http://www.webmd.com/digestive-disorders/exercise-curing-constipation-via-movement.

22. Schnelle, J. F., Leung, F. W., Rao, S. S., Beuscher, L., Keeler, E., Clift, J. W., Simmons, S. "A controlled trial of an intervention to improve urinary and fecal incontinence and constipation." *J Am Geriatr Soc.* 58, 8 (2010): 1504–1511.

23. Rodriquez, N. R. "Introduction to Protein Summit 2.0: continued exploration of the impact of high-quality protein on optimal health." *Am J Clin Nutr* 101, 6 (2105): 1317S–1319S.

24. Anderson, K. "Dietary regulation of cytochrome P450." *Ann Rev Nutr* 11, 4 (1991): 141–159.

25. Spaeth, G., Berg, R. D., Specian, R. D., Deitch, E. A. "Food without fiber promotes bacterial translocation from the gut." *Surgery* 108, 2 (1990):240–246.

26. Stresser, D. M., Bjeldanes, L. F., Bailey, G. S., Williams, D. E. "The anticarcinogen 3,3'-diindolylmethane is an inhibitor of cytochrome P-450." *J Biochem Toxicol* 10, 4 (1995):191–201.

27. National Institute Health, National Institute Environmental Health Science. "Indole-3-carbinol." Available at: http://ntp-server.niehs.nih.gov.

28. Jeffery, E. H. "Diet and Detoxification Enzymes." *The Proceedings from the 13th International Symposium of The Institute for Functional Medicine.* Supplement to *Alternative Therapies in Health and Medicine.* 2009: S98–S99.

29. Wong, G. Y., Bradlow, L., Sepkovic, D., et al. "Dose-ranging study of indole-3-carbinol for breast cancer prevention." *J Cell Biochem Suppl* 28–29 (1997): 111–116.

30. Michnovicz, J. J. "Increased estrogen 2-hydroxylation in obese women using oral indole-3-carbinol." *Int J Obes Relat Metab Disord* 22 (1998): 227–229.

31. Telang, N. T., Katdare, M., Bradlow, H. L., et al. "Inhibition of proliferation and modulation of estradiol metabolism: novel mechanisms for breast cancer prevention by the phytochemical indole-3-carbinol." *Proc Soc Exp Biol Med* 216 (1997): 246–252.

32. Jeffery, E.H. "Diet and Detoxification Enzymes." *The Proceedings from the 13th International Symposium of The Institute for Functional Medicine.* Supplement to *Alternative Therapies in Health and Medicine.* 2009: S98–S99.

33. Pantuck, E. J., Pantuck, C. B., Garland, W. A., Min, B. H., et al. "Stimulatory effect of Brussels sprouts and cabbage on human drug metabolism." *Clin Pharmacol Ther.* 25, 1 (1979): 88–95.

34. Prochaska, H. J., Santamaria, A. B., Talalay, P. "Rapid detection of inducers of enzymes that protect against carcinogens." *Proc Natl Acad Sci U S A.* 89,6 (1992): 2394–2398.

35. Ibid.

36. Nguyen, T., Rushmore. T.H., Pickett, C.B. "Transcriptional regulation of a rat liver glutathione S-transferase Ya subunit gene. Analysis of the antioxidant response element and its activation by the phorbol ester 12-O-tetradecanoylphorbol-13-acetate." *J Biol Chem* 269, 18 (1994): 13656–13662.

37. Nioi, P., Hayes, J. D. 'Contribution of NAD(P)H:quinone oxidoreductase 1 to protection against carcinogenesis, and regulation of its gene by the Nrf2 basic-region leucine zipper and the arylhydrocarbon receptor basic helix-loop-helix transcription factors.' *Mutat Res* 555, 1–2 (2004): 149–171.

38. Lee, J. S., Surh, Y. J. "Nrf2 as a novel molecular target for chemoprevention." *Cancer Lett.* 224, 2 (2005): 171–184.

39. Chan, L. M., Lowes, S., Hirst, B. H. "The ABCs of drug transport in intestine and liver: efflux proteins limiting drug absorption and bioavailability." *Eur J Pharm Sci* 21, 1 (2004): 25–51.

40. Hayashi, A., Suzuki, H., Itoh, K., Yamamoto, M., Sugiyama, Y. "Transcription factor Nrf2 is required for the constitutive and inducible expression of multidrug resistance-associated protein 1 in mouse embryo fibroblasts." *Biochem Biophys Res Commun* 310, 3 (2003): 824–829.

41. Moon, Y. J., Wang, X., Morris, M. E. "Dietary flavonoids: effects on xenobiotic and carcinogen metabolism." *Toxicol In Vitro.* 20, 2 (2006): 187–210.

42. Aggarwal, B. B., Ichikawa, H. "Molecular targets and anticancer potential of indole-3-carbinol and its derivatives." *Cell Cycle* 4, 9 (2005): 1201–1215.

43. Nho, C. W., Jeffery, E. "Crambene, a bioactive nitrile derived from glucosinolate hydrolysis, acts via the antioxidant response element to upregulate quinone reductase alone or synergistically with indole-3-carbinol." *Toxicol Appl Pharmacol.* 198, 1 (2004): 40–48.

44. Gescher, A. J., Sharma, R. A., Steward, W. P. "Cancer chemoprevention by dietary constituents: a tale of failure and promise." *Lancet Oncol* 2, 6 (2001): 371–379.

45. Ullmann, U., Haller, J., Decourt, J. P., et al. "A single ascending dose study of epigallocatechin gallate in healthy volunteers." *J Int Med Res.* 2003; 31(2):88–101.

46. Smith, B. "Organic foods versus supermarket foods: element levels," *J Appl Nutr.* 1993; 45(1):35–39.

47. Curl, C. L., Fenske, R. A., Elgethun, K. "Organophosphorus pesticide exposure of urban and suburban preschool children with organic and conventional diets." *Environ Health Perspect.* 2003; 111(3):377–382.

48. Westin, J. B., Richter, E. "The Israeli breast-cancer anomaly." *Ann N Y Acad Sci.* 1990; 609: 269–279.

49. Walker, C., Reamy, B. V. "Diets for cardiovascular disease prevention: what is the evidence?" *Am Fam Physician* 2009; 79(7): 571–578.

50. Mente, A., de Koning, L., Shannon, H.S., Anand, S.S. "A systematic review of

the evidence supporting a causal link between dietary factors and coronary heart disease." *Arch Intern Med* 2009;169(7):659–669.

51. Shai, I., Schwarzfuchs, D., Henkin, Y., et al. "Weight loss with a low-carbohydrate, Mediterranean, or low-fat diet." *N Engl J Med* 2008;359(3):229–241.

52. Agatston, A. *The South Beach Diet*. St. Martins Press; 2003.

53. Aude, Y.W., Agatston, A.S., Lopez-Jimenez, F., Lieberman, E.H., Marie Almon, Hansen, M., Rojas, G., Lamas, G.A., Hennekens, C.H. "The national cholesterol education program diet vs a diet lower in carbohydrates and higher in protein and monounsaturated fat: a randomized trial." *Arch Intern Med* 2004;164(19):2141–2146.

54. Atkins, R.C. *Dr. Atkins New Diet Revolution*. New York: Quill; 2002:47–55.

55. Brehm, B.J., Seeley, R.J., Daniels, S.R., et al. "A Randomized Trial Comparing a Very Low Carbohydrate Diet and a Calorie-Restricted Low Fat Diet on Body Weight and Cardiovascular Risk Factors in Healthy Women." *Journal of Clinical Endocrinology and Metabolism* 2003; 88(4):1617–1623.

56. Foster, G.D., Wyatt, H.R., Hill, J.O., et al. "A Randomized Trial of a Low-Carbohydrate Diet for Obesity." *New England Journal of Medicine* 2003; 348(21):2082–2090.

57. Tarantino, G., Citro, V., Finelli, C. "Hype or Reality: Should Patients with Metabolic Syndrome-related NAFLD be on the Hunter-Gatherer (Paleo) Diet to Decrease Morbidity?" *J Gastrointestin Liver Dis.* 2015 Sep;24(3):359–368.

58. Fontana, L., Meyer, T.E., Klein, S., Holloszy, J.O. "Long-term low-calorie low-protein vegan diet and endurance exercise are associated with low cardiometabolic risk." *Rejuvenation Res* 2007;10(2):225–234.

59. Key, T.J., Thorogood, M., Appleby, P.N., Burr. M.L. "Dietary habits and mortality in 11,000 vegetarians and health conscious people: results of a 17 year follow up." *BMJ* 1996;313(7060):775–779.

60. Cho, C.G., Kim, H.J., Chung, S.W., et al. "Modulation of glutathione and thioredoxin systems by calorie restriction during the aging process." *Exp Gerontol.* 2003;38(5):539–548.

61. Heilbronn, L.K., de Jonge, L., Frisard, M.I., et al. "Effect of 6-month calorie restriction on biomarkers of longevity, metabolic adaptation, and oxidative stress in overweight individuals: a randomized controlled trial." *JAMA.* 2006;295(13):1539–1548.

62. Jeffery, E.H. "Diet and Detoxification Enzymes." *The Proceedings from the 13th International Symposium of The Institute for Functional Medicine*. Supplement to *Alternative Therapies in Health and Medicine*. 2009: S98–S99.

63. Bennett, P. "Working Up the Toxic Patient: Practical Intervention and Treatment Strategies." *The Proceedings from the 13th International Symposium of The Institute for Functional Medicine*. Supplement to *Alternative Therapies in Health and Medicine*. 2009: S100–S106.

64. Michalsen, A., Weidenhammer, W., Melchart, D., Langhorst, J., Saha, J., Dobos, G. "Short term therapeutic fasting in the treatment of chronic pain and fatigue

syndromes—well-being and side effects with and without mineral supplements." [Article in German]. *Forsch Komplementarmed Klass Naturheilkd.* 2002;9(4):221–227.

65. Kimura, K.D., Tissenbaum, H.A., Liu, Y., Ruvkun, G. "daf-2, an insulin receptor-like gene that regulates longevity and diapause in Caenorhabditis elegans." *Science.* 1997;277(5328):942–946.

66. Greene, A.E., Todorova, M.T., Seyfried, T.N. "Perspectives on the metabolic management of epilepsy through dietary reduction of glucose and elevation of ketone bodies." *J Neurochem.* 2003;86(3):529–537.

67. Iwashige, K., Kouda, K., Kouda, J., et al. "Calorie restricted diet and urinary pentosidine in patients with rheumatoid arthritis." *J Physiol Anthropol Appl Human Sci.* 2004;23(1):19–24.

68. Lee, C., Weindruch, R. "Calorie intake, gene expression and aging." *In: 8th Symposium: Functional Medicine Approaches to Endocrine Disturbances of Aging.* Gig Harbor, WA: Institute for Functional Medicine; 2001.

69. Guarente, L., Kenyon, C. "Genetic pathways that regulate ageing in model organisms." *Nature.* 2000;408(6809):255–262.

70. Merry, B.J. "Oxidative stress and mitochondrial function with aging—the effects of calorie restriction." *Aging Cell.* 2004;3(1):7–12.

71. Lambert, A.J., Merry, B.J. "Effect of caloric restriction on mitochondrial reactive oxygen species production and bioenergetics: reversal by insulin." *Am J Physiol Regul Integr Comp Physiol.* 2004;286(1):R20–R21.

72. Mulas, M.F., Demuro, G., Mulas, C., et al. "Dietary restriction counteracts age-related changes in cholesterol metabolism in the rat." *Mech Ageing Dev.* 2005;126(6–7):648–654.

73. Sun, D., Krishnan, A., Su, J., et al. "Regulation of immune function by calorie restriction and cyclophosphamide treatment in lupus-prone NZB/NZW F1 mice." *Cell Immunol.* 2004;228(1):54–65.

74. Sanchez, A., Reese,r J.L., Lau, H.S., et al. "Role of sugars in human neutrophilic phagocytosis." *Am J Clin Nutr.* 1973;26(11):1180–1184.

75. Lamas, O., Martinez, J.A., Marti, A. "Energy restriction restores the impaired immune response in overweight (cafeteria) rats." *J Nutr Biochem.* 2004;15(7):418–425.

76. Mohanty, P., Hamouda, W., Garg, R., Aljida, A. Ghanim, H., Dandona, P. "Glucose challenge stimulates reactive oxygen species (ROS) generation by leucocytes." *J Clin Endocrinol Metab.* 2000;85(8):2970–2973.

77. Dandona, P., Mohanty, P., Hamouda, W., et al. "Inhibitory effect of a two day fast on reactive oxygen species (ROS) generation by leucocytes and plasma ortho-tyrosine and meta-tyrosine concentrations." *J Clin Endocrinol Metab.* 2001:86(6):2899–2902.

78. Bennett, P. "Working Up the Toxic Patient: Practical Intervention and Treatment Strategies." *The Proceedings from the 13th International Symposium of The Institute for Functional Medicine.* Supplement to *Alternative Therapies in Health and Medicine.* 2009: S100–S106.

79. Anderson, K. "Dietary regulation of cytochrome P450." *Annu Rev Nutr.* 1991;11(4):141–159.

80. Paganelli, R., Fagiolo, U., Cancian, M., et al. "Intestinal permeability in irritable bowel syndrome. Effect of diet and sodium cromoglycate administration." *Ann Allergy.* 1990;64(4):377–380.

81. Bennett, P. "Working Up the Toxic Patient: Practical Intervention and Treatment Strategies." *The Proceedings from the 13th International Symposium of The Institute for Functional Medicine.* Supplement to *Alternative Therapies in Health and Medicine.* 2009: S100–S106.

Chapter 8

1. Zouboulis, C.C., Makrantonaki, E. "Clinical aspects and molecular diagnostics of skin aging." *Clin Dermatol.* 2011;29:3–14.

2. Rittié, L., Fisher, G.J. "Natural and Sun-Induced Aging of Human Skin." *Cold Spring Harb Perspect Med.* 2015 Jan; 5(1): a015370.

3. Schmid, D., Muggl, R., Zülli, F. "Collagen glycation and skin aging." *C&T Manufacture Worldwide.* 2002:1–6.

4. Callaghan, T.M., Wilhelm, K.P. "A review of ageing and an examination of clinical methods in the assessment of ageing skin. Part I: Cellular and molecular perspectives of skin ageing." *Int J Cosmet Sci.* 2008 Oct;30(5):313–322.

5. DeGroot, J., Lafeber, F.P., Ban, R.A., TeKopple, J.M., Verzjil, N. "Glucosamine inhibits formation of advanced glycation endproducts in human articular cartilage: a mechanism for chondroprotection?" *49th Annual Meeting of the Orthopaedic Research Society.* Paper #0048; 2003:1 pg.

6. Gueniche, A., Castiel-Higounenc, I. "Efficacy of Glucosamine Sulphate in Skin Ageing: Results from an ex vivo Anti-Ageing Model and a Clinical Trial." *Skin Pharmacol Physiol.* 2017;30(1):36–41.

7. Kajimoto, O., Suguro, S., Takahashi, T. "Clinical Effects of Glucosamine Hydrochloride Diet for Dry Skin." *Nippon Shokuhin Kagaku Kogaku Kaishi* 2001;48(5):335–343.

8. Shimoda, H. et al. "Effect of cinnamoyl and flavonol glucosides derived from cherry blossom glowers on the production of advanced glycation end products (AGEs) and AGE-induced fibroblast apoptosis." *Phytotherapy Res.* 2011; 25: 1328–1335.

9. Yonei, et al. "Anti-glycation activity and safety of foods containing lingonberry extract and cherry blossom extract and chewable tablets containing citric acid and calcium.–A placebo-controlled randomized single-blind parallel group comparative study." *Anti-aging Med.* 2006; 10: 21–36.

10. Jean, D., Pouligon, M., Dalle, C. "Evaluation in vitro of AGE-crosslinks breaking ability of rosmarinic acid." *Glycative Stress Research* 2015; 2 (4): 204–207.

11. Miroliaei, M., Khazaei, S., Moshkelgosha, S., Shirvani, M. "Inhibitory effects of Lemon balm (Melissa officinalis, L.) extract on the formation of advanced glycation end products." *Food Chem.* 15 November 2011;129(2):267–271.

12. Yui, S., Fujiwara, S., Harada, K., Motoike-Hamura, M., Sakai, M., Matsubara, S., Miyazaki, K. "Beneficial effects of lemon balm leaf extract on in vitro glycation of proteins, arterial stiffness, and skin elasticity in healthy adults." *J Nutr Sci Vitaminol* (Tokyo). 2017;63(1):59–68.

13. Pacifici, G.M., Viani, A., Franch, M., Santerini, S., Temellini, A., Giuliani, L., Carra, M. "Conjugation pathways in liver disease." *Br J Clin Pharmac.* 1990;30:427–435.

14. "N-Acetyl-l-Cysteine monograph." *Alternative Medicine Review* 2000; 5(5); 467–471.

15. Zimet, I. "Acetylcysteine: A drug that is much more than a mucokinetic." *Biomed & Pharmacother* 1988;42:513–520.

16. De Flora, S., Grassi, C., Carat,i L. "Attenuation of influenza-like symptomatology and improvement of cell-mediated immunity with long-term N-acetylcysteine treatment." *Eur Respir J* 1997;10:1535–1541.

17. "N-Acetyl-l-Cysteine monograph." *Alternative Medicine Review* 2000; 5(5); 467–471.

18. Chan, M.Y. "The effect of berberine on bilirubin excretion in the rat." *Comp Med East West.* 1977 Summer;5(2):161–168.

19. Yin, J., Xing, H., Ye, J. "Efficacy of berberine in patients with type 2 diabetes mellitus." *Metabolism.* 2008 May;57(5):712–717.

20. Zhang, Y., Li, X., Zou, D., Liu, W., Yang, J., Zhu, N., Huo, L., Wang, M., Hong, J., Wu, P., Ren, G., Ning, G. "Treatment of type 2 diabetes and dyslipidemia with the natural plant alkaloid berberine." *J Clin Endocrinol Metab.* 2008 Jul;93(7):2559–2565.

21. Zhou, T., Chen, Y., Huang, C., Chen, G. "Caffeine induction of sulfotransferases in rat liver and intestine." *J Appl Toxicol.* 2012 Oct;32(10):804–809.

22. Maiti, S., Chen, X., Chen, G. "All-trans retinoic acid induction of sulfotransferases." *Basic Clin Pharmacol Toxicol.* 2005 Jan;96(1):44–53.

23. Walaszek, Z., Szemraj, J., Narog, M. "Metabolism, uptake, and excretion of a D-glucaric acid salt and its potential use in cancer prevention." *Cancer Detect Prev* 1997; 21:178–190.

24. Dwivedi, C., Heck, W.J., Downie, A.A., et al. "Effect of calcium glucarate on beta-glucuronidase activity and glucarate content of certain vegetables and fruits." *Biochem Med Metab Biol* 1990;43:83–92.

25. "Calcium-D-Glucarate monograph." *Altern Med Rev.* 2002;7(4):336–339.

26. "Curcuma longa (turmeric)." Monograph. *Altern Med Rev* 2001;6 Suppl: S62–S66.

27. Mortellini, R., Foresti, R., Bassi, R., Green, C.J. "Curcumin, an antioxidant and anti-inflammatory agent, induces heme oxygenase-1 and protects endothelial cells against oxidative stress." *Free Radic Biol Med* 2000;28:1303–1312.

28. Deshpande, U.R., Gadre, S.G., Raste, A.S., et al. "Protective effect of turmeric

(Curcuma longa L.) extract on carbon tetrachloride-induced liver damage in rats." *Indian J Exp Biol* 1998;36:573–577.

29. Makarova, S.I. "Human N-acetyltransferases and drug-induced hepato-toxicity." *Current Drug Metabolism.* 2008;9(6):538–545.

30. "Quercetin." *Alt Med Rev* 1998;3:140–143.

31. Shoskes, D.A., Zeitlin, S.I., Shahed, A., Rajfer, J. "Quercetin in men with category III chronic prostatitis: A preliminary prospective, double-blind, placebo-controlled trial." *Urol* 1999;54:960–963.

32. Chen, Y., Xiao, P., Ou-Yang, D.S., et al. "Simultaneous action of the flavonoid quercetin on cytochrome p450 (cyp) 1a2, cyp2a6, n-acetyltransferase and xanthine oxidase activity in healthy volunteers." *Clinical and Experimental Pharmacology.* 2009;36(8):828–833.

33. van Zandwijk, N. "N-acetylcysteine for lung cancer prevention." *Chest* 1995;107:1437–1441.

34. Morgan, L.R., Holdiness, M.R., Gillen, L.E. "N-acetylcysteine: its bioavailability and interaction with ifosfamide metabolites." *Semin Oncol* 1983;10:56–61.

35. Food and Nutrition Board, Institute of Medicine. "Pantothenic acid. Dietary Reference Intakes: Thiamin, Riboflavin, Niacin, Vitamin B6, Vitamin B12, Pantothenic Acid, Biotin, and Choline." Washington, D.C.: National Academy Press; 1998:357–373.

36. Crinnion, W.J. "Environmental Medicine, Part 2—Health Effects of and Protection from Ubiquitous Airborne Solvent Exposure." *Alternative Medicine Review* 2000; 5(2):133–143.

37. Hill, R.H., Jr, Ashley, D.L., Head, S.L., et al. "p-Dichlorobenzene exposure among 1,000 adults in the United States." *Arch Environ Health* 1995;50:277–280.

38. Yin, M., Ikejima. K., Artee,l G.E., Seabra, V., Bradford, B.U., Kono, H., Rusyn, I., Thurman, R.G. "Glycine accelerates recovery from alcohol-induced liver injury." *J Pharmacol Exp Ther.* 1998 Aug;286(2):1014–1019.

39. Wang, W.Y., Liaw, K.Y. "Effect of a taurine-supplemented diet on conjugated bile acids in biliary surgical patients." *JPEN J Parenter Enteral Nutr.* 1991 May–Jun;15(3):294–297.

40. Matsuyama, Y., Morita, T., Higuchi, M., Tsujii, T. "The effect of taurine administration on patients with acute hepatitis." *Prog Clin Biol Res* 1983;125:461–468.

41. Sacks, G.S. "Glutamine supplementation in catabolic patients." *Ann Pharmacother* 1999;33:348–354.

42. Ibid.

43. van der Hulst, R.R., van Kreel, B.K., von Meyenfeldt, M.F., et al. "Glutamine and the preservation of gut integrity." *Lancet* 1993;341:1363–1365.

44. Lerman, A., Burnett, J.C., Jr, Higano, S.T., et al. "Long-term L-arginine improves small-vessel coronary endothelial function in humans." *Circulation* 1998;97:2123–2128.

45. Wu, G., Bazer, F.W., Davis, T.A., Kim, S.W., Li, P., Marc Rhoads, J., Carey Satterfield, M., Smith, S.B., Spencer, T.E., Yin, Y. "Arginine metabolism and nutrition in growth, health and disease." *Amino Acids*. 2009 May;37(1):153–168.

46. Ozsoy, Y., Coskun, T., Yavu,z K., Ozbilgin, K., Var, A., Ozyurt, B. "The effects of L-arginine on liver damage in experimental acute cholestasis an immunohistochemical study." *HPB Surg.* 2011;2011:306069.

47. Ehren, I., Lundberg, J.O., Adolfsson, J., Wiklund, N.P. "Effects of L-arginine treatment on symptoms and bladder nitric oxide levels in patients with interstitial cystitis." *Urology* 1998;52:1026–1029.

48. Bucci, L.R., Hickson, J.F., Jr, Wolinsky, I, Pivarnik, J.M. "Ornithine supplementation and insulin release in bodybuilders." *Int J Sport Nutr* 1992;2:287–291.

49. Sugino, T., Shirai, T., Kajimoto, Y., and Kajimoto, O. "L-ornithine supplementation attenuates physical fatigue in healthy volunteers by modulating lipid and amino acid metabolism." *Nutr.Res.* 2008;28(11):738–743.

50. Vale, J.A., Meredith, T.J., Goulding, R. "Treatment of acetaminophen poisoning. The use of oral methionine." *Arch Intern Med* 1981;141:394–6.

51. Wu, W., Kang, S., Zhang, D. "Association of vitamin B6, vitamin B12 and methionine with risk of breast cancer: a dose-response meta-analysis." *Br J Cancer* 2013;109(7):1926–44.

52. Kuo, H. K., Sorond, F. A., Chen, J. H., Hashmi, A., Milberg, W. P., and Lipsitz, L. A. "The role of homocysteine in multisystem age-related problems: a systematic review." *J Gerontol.A Biol.Sci Med Sci* 2005;60(9):1190–1201.

53. "Dose-dependent effects of folic acid on blood concentrations of homocysteine: a meta-analysis of the randomized trials." *Am J Clin Nutr* 2005;82(4):806–812.

54. Potter, K., Hankey, G. J., Green, D. J., Eikelboom, J., Jamrozik, K., and Arnolda, L. F. "The effect of long-term homocysteine-lowering on carotid intima-media thickness and flow-mediated vasodilation in stroke patients: a randomized controlled trial and meta-analysis." *BMC.Cardiovasc.Disord* 2008;8:24.

55. Taylor, M.J., Carney, S.M., Goodwin, G.M., Geddes, J.R. "Folate for depressive disorders: systematic review and meta-analysis of randomized controlled trials." *J Psychopharmacol* 2004;18(2):251–6.

56. Gariballa, S., Forster, S. "Effects of dietary supplements on depressive symptoms in older patients: a randomised double-blind placebo-controlled trial." *Clin Nutr* 2007;26(5):545–51.

57. Hallert, C., Svensson, M., Tholstrup, J., Hultberg, B. "Clinical trial: B vitamins improve health in patients with coeliac disease living on a gluten-free diet." *Aliment Pharmacol Ther* 2009;29(8):811–6.

58. Coppen, A., Bailey, J. "Enhancement of the antidepressant action of fluoxetine by folic acid: a randomised, placebo controlled trial." *J Affect Dis* 2000;60:121–31.

59. Schwab, U., Torronen, A., Meririnne, E., Saarinen, M., Alfthan, G., Aro, A., and Uusitupa, M. "Orally administered betaine has an acute and dose-dependent

effect on serum betaine and plasma homocysteine concentrations in healthy humans." *J Nutr* 2006;136(1):34–38.

60. Rochat, F., Baumgartner, M., Jann, A., Rochat, C., Nielsen, G., Reuteler, G., Ballèvre, O. "Synergistic effect of prebiotics on human intestinal microflora." 2001—Ref Type: Personal Communication. In Meance S. Acacia gum (Fibregum™), a very well tolerated specific natural prebiotic having a wide range of food applications – Part 1. *AgroFOOD industry hi-tech.* 2004. January/February:24–28.

61. Cherbut, C., Michel, C., Raison, V., Kravtchenko, T.P., Meance, S. "Acacia Gum is a bifidogenic dietary fiber with high digestive tolerance in healthy humans." *Microbial Ecol Health Dis.* 2003; 15:43–50.

62. Wyatt, G.M., Bayliss, C.E., Holcroft, J.D. "A change in human faecal flora in response to inclusion of gum arabic in the diet." *Br J Nutr.* 1986; 55:261–266.

63. Baray, S. "Chapter 7: Acacia Gum." In Cho SS, Samuel P (Eds.). *Fiber Ingredients: Food Applications and Health Benefits.* Boca Raton, FL: CRC Press; 2009: 121–134.

64. Sokol, H., Pigneur, B., Watterlot, L., Lakhdari, O., Bermúdez-Humarán, L.G., Gratadoux, J.J., Blugeon S, Bridonneau C, Furet JP, Corthier G, Grangette C, Vasquez N, Pochart P, Trugnan G, Thomas, G., Blottière, H.M., Doré, J., Marteau, P., Seksik, P., Langella, P. "Faecalibacterium prausnitzii is an anti-inflammatory commensal bacterium identified by gut microbiota analysis of Crohn disease patients." *Proc Natl Acad Sci U S A.* 2008 Oct 28; 105(43):16731–16736.

65. Daguet, D., Pinheiro, I., Verhelst, A., Possemiers, S., Marzorati, M. "Acacia gum improves the gut barrier functionality in vitro." *Agro FOOD Industry Hi Tech.* July/August 2015;26(4):29–33.

66. Daguet, D., Pinheiro, I., Verhelst, A., Possemiers, S., and Marzorati, M. "Arabinogalactan and fructooligosaccharides improve the gut barrier function in distinct areas of the colon in the Simulator of the Human Intestinal Microbial Ecosystem." *J Fuct Foods.* 2016;20:369–379.

67. Eliaz, I. "Modified citrus pectin (MCP) in the treatment of cancer." Paper presented at: The American Chemical Society Annual Meeting; Philadelphia, PA; 2004

68. Zhao, Z.Y., et al. 2008. "The Role of Modified Citrus Pectin as an Effective Chelator of Lead in Children Hospitalized with Toxic Lead Levels." *Altern Ther Health Med* 14(4):34–38.

69. Eliaz, I., Weil, E., Wilk, B. "Integrative Medicine and the Role of Modified Citrus Pectin/Alginates in Heavy Metal Chelation and Detoxification—Five Case Reports." *Forsch Komplementärmed* 2007;14:358–364.

70. Patrick, L. "Mercury Toxicity and Antioxidants: Part I: Role of Glutathione and alpha-Lipoic Acid in the Treatment of Mercury Toxicity." *Altern Med Rev* 2002;7(6):458.

71. Ballatori, N., Lieberman, M.W., Wang, W. "N-Acetylcysteine as an Antidote in Methylmercury Poisoning." *Environ Health Prect* 1998;106:267–271.

72. Kelly, G.S. "Clinical Applications of N-acetylcysteine." *Alt Med Rev* 1998;3(2):114–127.

73. Abdalla, F.H., Bellé, L.P., De Bona, K.S., Bitencourt, P.E., Pigatto, A.S., Moretto, M.B. "Allium sativum L. extract prevents methyl mercury-induced cytotoxicity in peripheral blood leukocytes (LS)." *Food Chem Toxicol* 2010;48(1):417–421.

74. Cha, C-W. "A study on the effect of garlic to the heavy metal poisoning of rat." *J Korean Med Sci* 1987;2(4):213–223.

75. Li. Y-F., Dong, Z., Chen, C., et al. "Organic selenium supplementation increases mercury excretion and decreases oxidative damage in long-term mercury-exposed residents from Wanshan, China." *Environmental Science & Technology.* 2012;46(20):11313–11318.

Chapter 9

1. Krop, J. "Chemical sensitivity after intoxication at work with solvents: response to sauna therapy." *J Altern Complement Med.* 1998;4(1):77–86.

2. Kilburn, K.H., Warsaw, R.H., Shields, M.G. "Neurobehavioral dysfunction in firemen exposed to polycholorinated biphenyls (PCBs): possible improvement after detoxification." *Arch Environ Healt.* 1989;44(6):345–350.

3. Crinnon, W. "Components of Practical Clinical Detox Programs—Sauna as a Therapeutic Tool." *The Proceedings from the 13th International Symposium of The Institute for Functional Medicine.* Supplement to *Alternative Therapies in Health and Medicine.* 2009:S154–S156.

4. Cohn, J.R., Emmet, E.A. "The excretion of trace metals in human sweat." *Ann Clin Lab Sci.* 1978;8(4):270–275.

5. Crinnon, W. "Components of Practical Clinical Detox Programs—Sauna as a Therapeutic Tool." *The Proceedings from the 13th International Symposium of The Institute for Functional Medicine.* Supplement to *Alternative Therapies in Health and Medicine.* 2009:S154–S156.

6. Mooventhan, A., Nivethitha, L. "Scientific evidence-based effects of hydrotherapy on various systems of the body." *N Am J Med Sci.* 2014 May;6(5): 199–209.

7. Heywood, A. "A trial of the Bath waters: the treatment of lead poisoning." *Med Hist Suppl.* 1990;10:82–101.

8. Siems, W.G., van Kuijk, F.J., Maass, R., Brenke, R. "Uric acid and glutathione levels during short-term whole body cold exposure." *Free Radic Biol Med* 1994;16(3):299–305.

9. Kuhn, G., Buhring, M. "Physical medicine and quality of life: design and results of a study on hydrotherapy." *Comp Ther Med* 1995;3:138–141.

10. Stener-Victorin, E., Kruse-Smidje, C., Jung K. "Comparison between electro-acupuncture and hydrotherapy, both in combination with patient education and patient education alone, on the symptomatic treatment of osteoarthritis of the hip." *Clin J Pain* 2004;20(3):179–185.

11. Foley, A., Halbert, J., Hewitt, T., Crotty, M. "Does hydrotherapy improve strength and physical function in patients with osteoarthritis—a randomized controlled trial comparing a gym based and a hydrotherapy based strengthening programme." *Ann Rheum Dis* 2003;62(12):1162–1167.

12. Michalsen, A., Ludtke, R., Buhring, M,. Spahn, G., Langhorst, J., Dobos, G.J. "Thermal hydrotherapy improves quality of life and hemodynamic function in patients with chronic heart failure." *Am Heart J* 2003;146(4):728–733.

13. Kesiktas, N., Pake, N., Erdogan, N., Gulsen, G., Bicki, D., Yilmaz, H. "The use of hydrotherapy for the management of spasticity." *Neurorehabil Neural Repair.* 2004;18(4):268–273.

14. Cassar, M-P. "Massage for detoxification." Pacific College of Oriental Medicine. Retrieved August 21, 2018 from https://www.pacificcollege.edu/news/blog/2014/07/15/massage-detoxification.

15. Xujian, Shao. "Effect of massage and temperature on the permeability of initial lymphatics." *Lymphology* 1990;23: 48–50.

16. "Report on the Proceedings of a Summit on New Directions for Chelation Therapy." *Townsend Letter* August / September 2013. Retrieved September 29, 2018 from http://www.townsendletter.com/AugSept2013/chelationsummit0813.html.

About the Authors

Earl Mindell, RPh, MH, PhD, is a registered pharmacist and college educator. He is also the award-winning author of over twenty best-selling books, including *Earl Mindell's New Vitamin Bible*. He has been inducted into the California Pharmacists Association's Hall of Fame and awarded the President's Citation for Exemplary Service from Bastyr University. He is on the board of directors of the California College of Natural Medicine and has been a member of the Dean's Professional Advisory Group at Chapman University School of Pharmacy. He is also an associate professor at Chapman University.

Gene Bruno, MS, MHS, is professor of nutraceutical science and provost at Huntington University of Health Sciences. He holds graduate degrees in both nutrition and herbal medicine, and is a registered herbalist with the American Herbalists Guild. For forty years, he has educated healthcare professionals and others in nutrition, herbal medicine, and nutraceutical sciences. He has written numerous articles on nutrition, herbal medicine, nutraceuticals, and integrative health issues for many magazines and peer-reviewed publications. He has also contributed chapters to many nutraceutical textbooks and is the author of *A Guide to Complementary Treatments for Diabetes*.

Index

Acacia gum, 160–161
Acetone, 71
Acetylation, 54, 152
Adenosine triphosphate (ATP), 64–65, 70
Air, fresh, 118
Alanine aminotransferase (ALAT), 35
Albumin, 7, 34
Albumin/globulin (A/G) ratio, 35
Alcohol, 124
Alkaline phosphatase (ALP), 35
Alpha-lipoic acid, 162
Amino acid conjugation, 54, 153–155
Amino acids, 7, 75–77
Ammonia, 32
Anemia
   microcytic, 16
   pernicious, 16
   sickle cell, 9, 19
Antibodies, 8
   A, 9
   B, 9
Antigens, 8
   A, 9
   B, 9
   and blood type, 10
   Rh factor, 10–11
Antioxidants, 16
Aorta, 23
Arginine, 155
Arteries, 21
Asparate aminotransferase (ASAT), 36

Atherogenic diet, 88
Atherosclerosis, 28, 74, 88
Atkins diet, 138
Atkins, Robert, 138

B cells, 13
Bacteremia, 133
Basic metabolic panel, 29–33
Basophils, 12–13
Berberine, 148
Betaine, 157
Bicarbonate (HCO3), 31–32
Bile, 23, 74
Bilirubin, 35
Biomarkers, 29
Blood
   amount of, in the human body, 5
   composition of, 5–14
   disorders, genetic, 19
   donor guide, 11
   filtration, 23
   influences on, 14–20
   pathways of the, 22–24
   sugar, 29. See also Glucose.
   tests, 25–45
   types, 10–11
   urea nitrogen (BUN), 32
   vessels, 21–24
Bone marrow, 8, 12–13, 19, 37
Breakdown products of protein metabolism, 51
Breathing, 121–123
BUN/creatinine ratio, 33

Caffeine, 148–149
Calcitonin, 30
Calcium, 29–30, 82
Calcium D-glucarate, 150
Caloric restriction, 139–142
Cancer, 89–91
Capillaries, 21–22
Capsaicin, 101
Carbohydrates, 65–69
Carbon dioxide (CO_2), 31–32
Carbonic acid (H_2CO_3), 31
Carson, Rachel, 18
Cellular respiration, 31
Chelation therapy, 169–170
Cherry blossom extract, 145
Chloride, 31, 83–84
Cholesterol, 27–28, 57, 64, 68, 72, 74
  high-density lipoprotein (HDL),
    17, 26–29, 73
  low-density lipoprotein (LDL),
    17, 26–28, 71
  total, 17, 26–28
  very low-density lipoprotein
    (VLDL), 27–28
Choline, 82
Chromium, 82
Chromosomes, 18, 20
Chronic kidney disease (CKD), 33
Cigarettes, 124
Circulatory system, 22–24
Collagen, 80
Complete blood count (CBC) panel,
  36–39
Constipation, 128–130, 132
Cooking techniques, 101–102
Copper, 15, 82
Coronary artery disease, 29
Cortisol, 43
C-reactive protein (CRP), 26, 44
Creatine, 32
Creatinine, 32
Curcumin, 151–152
Cytoplasm, 13
Cytotoxic T cells, 13

Dairy, 98–99
Dehydroepiandrosterone (DHEA),
  39–40

Dehydroepiandrosterone sulfate
  (DHEAS), 40
Detoxification
  heavy metal, 161–164
  intestines, 55–56, 158–161
  kidney, 146
  liver, 52–55, 146–158
  skin, 144–146
Detoxification mechanisms, support-
  ing, 133–136, 143–164
Detoxification guide, 57–58
D-glucaric acid, 150
Diabetes, 29, 66–67, 92–93
Diet
  atherogenic, 88
  Atkins, 138
  choosing, 136–142
  detoxification and, 132–136
  influence of, on blood, 15–17,
    106–108
  low-carb/high-protein diet,
    66–67, 106
  Mediterranean, 72, 89, 91, 107,
    136–137
  MyPlate, 107
  Okinawan, 89
  Paleo, 138
  Plant-based, 108, 139
  South Beach, 137–138
  toxic buildup and, 127–131
Dietary supplements, 143–164
Dipeptide, 7
Diverticula, 69
Diverticulitis, 69
DNA, 18
Drug and food interactions, 131
Drugs, 124

Edema, 34
Electrolytes, 30, 82
Endogenous toxins. *See* Toxins,
  internal.
Environment, influence of, on blood,
  18
Enzymes, 15
Eosinophils, 12
Epigenetics, 20
Erythrocytes. *See* Red blood cells.

Erythropoietin, 37
Estradiol (E2), 40
Estriol (E3), 40
Estrogen, 40
Estrone (E1), 40
Exercise, 116–117
Exogenous toxins. *See* Toxins, external.

Fasting, 139–142
Fat, 70
    saturated, 71–72
    unsaturated, 72–73
    See also Lipids; Triglycerides;
    Cholesterol.
Fermentation, 68
Fiber, dietary, 67–68
    insoluble, 68–69
    soluble, 68
Fibrinogen, 7
Folic acid, 15
Free radicals, 16
Fructose, 29, 65
Fruit, 94–95, 103

Galactose, 29, 65
Gamma delta T cells, 13
Gamma-glutamyl transferase (GGT),
    36
Garlic extract, 163
Genetics, influence of, on blood,
    18–20
Genes, 18
Globulin, 7, 34
    alpha, 34
    beta, 34
    gamma, 8
Glomerular filtration rate (GFR), 33
Glucosamine hydrochloride,
    144–145
Glucose, 29, 65–66, 70
Glucose tolerance factor (GTF), 82
Glucuronidation, 54, 149
Glutamine, 154–155
Glutathione conjugation, 54–55,
    150–152
Glutathione peroxidase, 84
Glycation, 144
Glycemic index (GI), 92–93

Glycine, 153–154
Glycogen, 65
Grains, 93–94, 103

Heart chambers
    left ventricle, 22–23
    right ventricle, 22
Heart disease, 88–89
Heavy metals, 47–48
Hematocrit, 37
Heme, 19
Hemochromatosis, 19
Hemoglobin, 8–9, 37
Hemophilia, 19
Hepatic function panel, 33
Hepatic portal vein, 23
Herbs, 100–101
Heterocylic amines (HCAs), 101
High blood sugar, 29
Hippocampus, 43
Histamine, 12–13
Homocysteine, 26, 43–44, 157
Hormones, 39–43
Hydrotherapy, 166–167
Hyperchromia, 38
Hyperexcitability, 41
Hyperglycemia. *See* High blood
    sugar.
Hyperplasia, 40
Hyperthyroidism, 42
Hypertriglyceridemia, 26
Hypochromia, 38
Hypoglycemia. *See* Low blood
    sugar.
Hypothyroidism, 42
Hypoxemia, 112
Hypoxia, 112
    anemic, 114
    histoxic, 115
    hypoxemic, 112–113
    stagnant, 114–115

Immunoglobulin. *See* Globulin,
    gamma.
Insulin, 29
Iodine, 83
Iron, 15, 83
Ischemia, 140

Ketones, 70–71
Ketosis, 70

Landsteiner, Karl, 10
Laughter, 123
Leaky gut syndrome, 130
Legumes, 97, 104
Lemon balm, 145–146
Leukemia, 19
Leukocytes. *See* White blood cells.
Lipid panel, 25–26
Lipids, 26, 70
Lipoprotein, 27, 74
Low blood sugar, 29
Low-carb/high-protein diet, 66–67, 106
Lymphocytes, 13

Macrocytosis, 38
Macronutrients, 64–77
Macrophages, 13
Magnesium, 44–45, 83
Manganese, 83
Massage, 123, 167–168
Maximal oxygen consumption, 17
Mean corpuscular hemoglobin (MCH), 38
Mean corpuscular hemoglobin concentration (MCHC), 38
Mean corpuscular volume (MCV), 38
Meat, 96–97
Meditation, 123, 170–171
Mediterranean diet, 72, 89, 91, 107, 136–137
Melanin, 82
Methemoglobinemia, 114
Methionine, 43, 156
Methylation, 55, 155–157
Microbial compounds, 50
Microcytosis, 38
Micronutrients, 77–78, 103–104
Milk thistle, 150–151
Minerals, 81–84
    major, 81
    trace, 81
Modified alginate complex, 162
Modified citrus pectin, 162
Monocytes, 13

MyPlate diet, 107

N-Acetylcysteine (NAC), 147–148, 152–153, 163
N-Acetyltransferase (NAT), 152
Natural killer cells, 13
Neurotransmitter, 82
Neutrophils, 12
Nitrogen, 32
Nutrient absorption, 63–64
Nuts, 97–98, 104

Okinawan diet, 89
Omega-3 fatty acids, 73
Omega-6 fatty acids, 73
Organic food, 104–106, 137
Ornithine, 155
Osteoporosis, 30
Oxygen
    increasing, levels, 116–124
    influence of, on blood, 109–124
    therapy, 120–121

Paleo diet, 138
Pantothenic acid, 153
Parathyroid hormone (PTH), 30
Pathogen, 8
Peptide, 7
Peripheral artery disease, 28
pH
    acidic, 14–15
    alkaline, 14–15
    balance, 14–15
    scale, 14
Phosphorus, 82
Physical Activity Guidelines for Americans, 17
Physical activity, influence of, on blood, 17
Physiological altitude, 113
Plant stanols, 97
Plant-based diet, 108, 139
Plasma, 6–8
    proteins, 7–8
Platelets, 13–14, 38–39
Polycyclic aromatic hydrocarbons, 102
Polycystic ovary syndrome, 40
Potassium, 30, 83–84

Porphyria, 19
Prayer, 123
Prebiotics, 160–161
Pregnancy eclampsia, 34
Probiotics, 68, 158–160
Progesterone, 41
Progestins, 41
Prostate-specific antigen (PSA), 42
Protein, 7–8, 74–75, 96–98, 104. *See also* Total protein count.
Pulmonary artery, 21
Pulmonary circulation, 22
Pulmonary vein, 21

Quercetin, 152

RBC antigens, 9–11
Red blood cells (RBCs), 8–11, 36–37
Regulatory T cells, 13
Retinoic acid, 149
Rh factor antigen. *See* Antigen, Rh factor.
Rh negative, 10–11
Rh positive, 10–11

Sauna therapy, 165–166
Seeds, 97–98, 104
Selenium, 84, 163–164
Serotonin, 13
Sickle cell anemia. *See* Anemia, sickle cell.
Silent Spring (Carson), 18
Sodium, 30–31, 83–84
South Beach Diet, 137–138
Spices, 100-101
Stroke, 91–92
Sulfation, 55, 147–149
Sulfotransferases (SULTs), 148–149
Systemic circulation, 22

T cells, 13
T helper cells, 13
T lymphocytes, 84
Taurine, 154
Testosterone, 41
    bound, 41
    free, 41
    total, 41
Thalassemia, 19

Thrombocytes. *See* Platelets.
Thrombocythemia, 39
Thyroid gland, 42
Thyroid-stimulating hormone (TSH), 42
Thyroxine (T$_4$), 42
Total protein count, 34
Toxins
    eliminating, from the body, 51–59
    external, 47–49
    internal, 49–51
Triglycerides, 26–28, 73–74
Triiodothyronine (T$_3$), 42
Tripeptide, 7, 54
Turmeric, 151–152

Umbilical artery, 21
Umbilical vein, 21
Universal donor, 11
Universal recipient, 11
Urea, 32
Ureter, 23
Urethra, 23
Urine, 23

Vasodilation, 115
Vegan. *See* Plant-based, diet.
Vegetables, 95, 103
    leafy green, 103
Vegetarian. *See* Plant-based, diet.
Veins, 21
Villi, 63
Vitamin A, 79, 149
Vitamin B$_5$, 153
Vitamin B$_6$, 156–157
Vitamin B$_9$, 156–157
Vitamin B$_{12}$, 16, 79, 156–157
Vitamin B-complex, 79–80
Vitamin C, 16, 79–80
Vitamin D, 44, 71, 74, 79–80
Vitamin E, 79–80
Vitamin K, 71, 79–80
Vitamins, 78–81
    fat-soluble, 79
    water-soluble, 79

Water, 6, 77, 99–100, 118
White blood cells (WBCs), 12, 39

Zinc, 84

Your Blood Never Lies

How to Read a Blood Test
for a Longer, Healthier Life

James B. LaValle, RPh, CCN

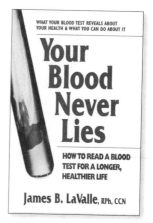

A standard blood test shows how well
the kidneys and liver are functioning,
the potential for heart disease, and a
host of other vital health markers. But
most of us cannot decipher these results
ourselves or even formulate the right
questions to ask—or we couldn't, until
now. In simple language, Dr. LaValle explains all of the information found on these forms, making it understandable and
accessible so that you can look at the results yourself and know
the significance of each marker.

$16.95 US • 368 pages • 6 x 9-inch paperback • ISBN 978-0-7570-0350-9

The Acid-Alkaline Food Guide
SECOND EDITION

A Quick Reference to Foods &
Their Effect on pH Levels

Susan E. Brown, PhD, and Larry Trivieri, Jr.

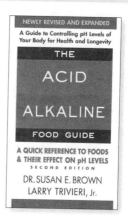

The importance of acid-alkaline
balance to good health is no secret.
The Acid-Alkaline Food Guide was
designed as an easy-to-follow guide to
the most common foods that influence
your body's pH level. Now in its second edition, this bestseller
has been expanded to include many more domestic and
international foods. Updated information also explores
(and refutes) the myths about pH balance and diet, and guides
you to supplements that can help you achieve a pH level that
supports greater well-being.

$8.95 US • 224 pages • 4 x 7-inch paperback • ISBN 978-0-7570-0393-6

What You Must Know About Vitamins, Minerals, Herbs and So Much More

SECOND EDITION

Pamela Wartian Smith, MD

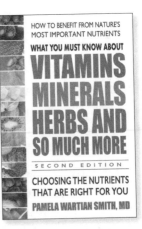

What You Must Know About Vitamins, Minerals, Herbs and So Much More guides you in restoring and maintaining health through the wise use of nutrients. Part One discusses the individual nutrients necessary for well-being, Part Two offers nutritional programs for a wide variety of health concerns, and Part Three presents supplementation plans. Whether you want to preserve good health or overcome a medical condition, this book will give you the information you need to make the best nutritional choices possible.

$16.95 US • 464 pages • 6 x 9-inch paperback • ISBN 978-0-7570-0471-1

Magnificent Magnesium

Your Essential Key to a Healthy Heart & More

Dennis Goodman, MD

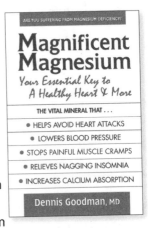

Despite the development of many "breakthrough" drugs, heart disease remains the number-one killer of Americans. In *Magnificent Magnesium*, world-renowned cardiologist Dr. Dennis Goodman shines a spotlight on magnesium, the mineral that can maximize your heart health without causing side effects. The author first establishes a firm foundation for understanding heart disease. Next, he details magnesium's astounding heart-healthy benefits, as well as the additional advantages it provides for other diseases. Finally, he offers clear guidelines on how to select and use this mineral to greatest effect.

$14.95 US • 192 pages • 6 x 9-inch paperback • ISBN 978-0-7570-0391-2

**For more information on our books,
visit our website at www.squareonepublishers.com**